Nicole Verhaar

Pharmacological preconditioning and ischaemic postconditioning in experimental jejunal ischaemia in horses

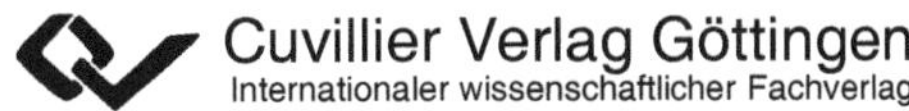

Bibliografische Information der Deutschen Nationalbibliothek
Die Deutsche Nationalbibliothek verzeichnet diese Publikation in der Deutschen Nationalbibliografie; detaillierte bibliographische Daten sind im Internet über http://dnb.d-nb.de abrufbar.
1. Aufl. - Göttingen: Cuvillier, 2021
Zugl.: Hannover (TiHo), Univ., Diss., 2021

Nonnenstieg 8, 37075 Göttingen
Telefon: 0551-54724-0
Telefax: 0551-54724-21
www.cuvillier.de

1. Auflage, 2021
Gedruckt auf umweltfreundlichem, säurefreiem Papier aus nachhaltiger Forstwirtschaft.

ISBN 978-3-7369-7433-3
eISBN 978-3-7369-6433-4

University of Veterinary Medicine Hannover

Clinic for Horses

Pharmacological preconditioning and ischaemic postconditioning in experimental jejunal ischaemia in horses

---

Thesis

Submitted in partial fulfilment of the requirements for the degree

Doctor of Philosophy (PhD)

Awarded by the University of Veterinary Medicine Hannover

Nicole Verhaar

Born in Amsterdam, The Netherlands

Hannover, Germany 2021

Supervision group: Prof. Dr. Sabine Kästner
Prof. Dr. Marion Hewicker-Trautwein
Prof. Dr. Christiane Pfarrer
Prof. Dr. Anja Kipar

1st evaluation: **Prof. Dr. Sabine Kästner**
Small Animal Clinic, University of Veterinary Medicine Hannover
Bünteweg 9, 30559 Hannover

Prof. Dr. Marion Hewicker-Trautwein
Institute for Pathology, University of Veterinary Medicine Hannover
Bünteweg 17, 30559 Hannover

Prof. Dr. Christiane Pfarrer
Institute for Anatomy, University of Veterinary Medicine Hannover
Bischofsholer Damm 15, 30176 Hannover

Prof. Dr. Anja Kipar
Institute of Veterinary Pathology, Vetsuisse Faculty
University of Zurich
Winterthurerstrasse 268, CH-8057 Zürich

2nd Evaluation: **Prof. Dr. Christiane Herden**
Institute for Veterinary Pathology
Justus-Liebig-Universität Gießen, Fachbereich Veterinärmedizin
Frankfurter Str. 96, 35392 Gießen

Date of final exam: 13 April 2021

Funding

- This study was partially funded by a research grant from the European College of Veterinary Surgeons (2019 LA) and Stiftung ProPferd (2019/04).

Sections of this thesis that have been published previously

Publications in peer-reviewed journals

- N Verhaar, C Pfarrer, S Neudeck, K König, K Rohn, L Twele, S Kästner; Preconditioning with lidocaine and xylazine in experimental equine jejunal ischaemia. *Equine Veterinary Journal 2021 53 (1) 125-133; doi.org/10.1111/evj.13251*
- N Verhaar, G Breves, M Hewicker-Trautwein, C Pfarrer, K Rohn, M Burmester, N Schnepel, S Neudeck, L Twele, S Kästner; The effect of ischaemic postconditioning on mucosal integrity and function in equine jejunal ischaemia. *Equine Veterinary Journal 2021 00:1-11; doi.org/10.1111/evj.13450*
- N Verhaar, N de Buhr, M von Köckritz-Blickwede, M Hewicker-Trautwein, C Pfarrer, H Schulze, S Kästner; Ischaemic postconditioning reduces apoptosis in experimental jejunal ischaemia in horses. *BMC Veterinary Research 2021 17:175;* doi.org/10.1186/s12917-021-02877-y

Abstracts at scientific meetings

- N Verhaar, C Pfarrer, S Neudeck, K König, K Rohn, L Twele, S Kästner; The effect of lidocaine and xylazine in an experimental model of equine jejunal ischaemia. *European College of Veterinary Surgeons (ECVS) Scientific meeting 2019, Budapest, Hungary*
- L Twele, S Neudeck, N Verhaar, J Reiners, S Kästner; Comparison of the cardiovascular effects of lidocaine or xylazine constant-rate infusion (CRI) in horses anaesthetized with isoflurane. *Association of Veterinary Anaesthetists (AVA) Scientific meeting, 2019, Bristol, United Kingdom*
- N. Verhaar, C. Pfarrer, S. Neudeck. K. König, K. Rohn, L. Twele, S. Kästner; The effect of xylazine and lidocaine on inflammation during small intestinal ischaemia in horses. *DVG 4th International Equine Congress (2020), Berlin, Germany*

This thesis is dedicated to my parents
for all their loving support
and encouragement

TABLE OF CONTENTS

List of Abbreviations

ANOVA	Analysis of Variance
CMA	Cranial mesenteric artery
CK	Creatinine-Kinase
DMSO	Dimethyl-sulfoxide
HIF	Hypoxia Inducible Factor
HSP	Heat Shock Protein
IPC	Ischaemic Preconditioning
IPoC	Ischaemic Postconditioning
I/R	Ischaemia / Reperfusion
LDH	Lactate-Dehydrogenase
Laser	Light amplification by stimulated emission of radiation
MAC	Minimal Alveolar Concentration
MDA	Malondialdehyde
MPO	Myeloperoxidase
mPTP	Mitochondrial Permeability Transition Pores
NOS	Nitric Oxide Synthase
PPC	Pharmacological Preconditioning
PPoC	Pharmacological Postconditioning
RC	Remote Conditioning
SOD	Superoxide Dismutase
TJ	Tight Junction
TUNEL	Terminal deoxynucleotidyl transferase dUTP Nick-End Labelling

1. Summary

Nicole Verhaar

Pharmacological preconditioning and ischaemic postconditioning in experimental jejunal ischaemia in horses

Strangulating obstruction of the small intestine in the horse is associated with a high mortality rate. Although many intestinal lesions can be treated surgically by intestinal resection, more effective strategies are needed to decrease the occurrence of complications related to the intestinal segments that are not amenable to resection. Preconditioning represents an increasingly popular treatment modality for ischaemia-reperfusion (I/R) injury in human medicine, and is predominantly applied in cardiology. It refers to the activation of intrinsic cell survival programmes after exposure to mild ischaemic stimuli or pharmacologic agents prior to an ischaemic event. Some of the protective mechanisms exerted by preconditioning may also be activated after ischaemia, as the blood supply is being reinstated. This principle of ischaemic postconditioning (IPoC) is defined as delayed reperfusion, and is performed by the repeated re-occlusion of the blood supply immediately after an ischaemic event. These treatment strategies have been shown to significantly ameliorate ischaemia reperfusion injury in different tissues and species.

The aim of this study was to determine the effect of pharmacological preconditioning (PPC) and IPoC on small intestinal I/R injury in horses. To achieve this, we performed two randomized controlled experimental in vivo studies. In both experiments, segmental jejunal ischaemia with 90% flow reduction was implemented in horses under general anaesthesia. In the first study, the horses were pharmacologically preconditioned with either xylazine (n=5) or lidocaine (n=5). A historical, untreated control group (n=5) was used for group comparison. In the second study, investigating IPoC, the test group (n=7) was subjected to delayed reperfusion by repeated clamping of the mesenteric vessels after ischaemia. In the control group (n=7), the jejunum was reperfused without further intervention. In both studies, the intestinal microperfusion and tissue oxygen saturation were measured using laser Doppler flowmetry and white light spectrophotometry. Furthermore, intestinal tissue samples were collected for histology, immunohistochemical staining, and biochemical analysis. Comparison of these variables between the groups and time points were performed using a 2-way repeated measures ANOVA with appropriate post-hoc tests ($p < 0.05$.). For ordinal and not normally distributed data, Mann-Whitney or Kruskal-Wallis tests were used for group comparison, and a Friedman test for comparisons of the time points within the groups.

As described in the first manuscript, PPC with lidocaine and xylazine did not ameliorate the I/R induced histomorphological changes. Xylazine treatment did result in a lower apoptotic cell count after ischaemia, and fewer inflammatory cells in the mucosa and serosa after reperfusion compared to the control group. Lidocaine treatment had no effect on I/R induced apoptosis and inflammation compared to the other groups.

In the IPoC study, as reported in the second and third manuscript, postconditioning clamping of the mesenteric vessels effectively reduced the intestinal microperfusion during all clamping cycles, yet affected tissue oxygenation only during the first cycle. The mesentery and its vessels did not show any signs of increased tissue damage after IPoC compared to the mesentery of the control group. Postconditioning resulted in reduced epithelial denudation, a lower apoptotic cell count and decreased paracellular permeability after reperfusion compared to the control group. The majority of the other tested variables for histomorphometry, cell death, inflammation, oxidative stress, and heat shock response were significantly affected by the ischaemia model as indicated by differences between the time points. However, none of these I/R responses were modified by IPoC.

The fourth manuscript describes the hypoxia inducible factor (HIF) response in this experimental model including the effect of IPoC. Significant changes were seen in mucosal HIF-1α immunoreactivity after reperfusion compared to pre-ischaemia, yet HIF-2α did not show any progression during ischaemia or reperfusion. These results suggest that transcription factor HIF-1α and not factor HIF-2α plays a role in the intestinal response to ischaemia. No effect of IPoC could be found on the immunoreactivity patterns of these hypoxia inducible factors.

In conclusion, xylazine PPC was associated with a reduction in apoptotic and inflammatory cells, indicating a beneficial effect of xylazine on intestinal I/R injury. These results would support the use of xylazine in sedative analgesia and anaesthetic protocols for horses with strangulating small intestinal lesions. IPoC was feasible and safe to perform, and the results suggest a possible protective effect of IPoC on I/R induced mucosal injury. Several potential mechanisms such as oxidative stress levels, HIF and heat shock response were investigated, yet were not affected by IPoC. The concept of IPoC may be a feasible therapeutic strategy with potential benefits for the colic patient; however, the exact mechanism and its long-term effects need to be elucidated before this can be implemented in clinical cases.

2. Zusammenfassung

Nicole Verhaar

Pharmakologische Präkonditionierung und ischämische Postkonditionierung in experimenteller Dünndarmischämie beim Pferd

Dünndarmstrangulationen beim Pferd sind mit einer hohen Mortalitätsrate assoziiert. Obwohl viele Darmläsionen mittels einer Dünndarmresektion chirurgisch therapiert werden können, bedarf es zusätzlicher Strategien zur Reduktion von Komplikationen im Zusammenhang mit Darmsegmenten, die nicht reseziert werden können. Präkonditionierung stellt eine zunehmend populäre Maßnahme zur Behandlung von Ischämie-Reperfusionsschäden (IRS) in der Humanmedizin dar, die vor allem im Bereich der Kardiologie eingesetzt wird. Unter Präkonditionierung wird die Aktivierung protektiver, intrinsischer Zellreaktionen infolge ischämischer oder pharmakologischer Stimuli vor dem eigentlichen Vorgang der Ischämie verstanden. Manche dieser, im Rahmen der Präkonditionierung auftretenden, protektiven Mechanismen können auch nach der Ischämie, zum Zeitpunkt der Wiederherstellung der Blutversorgung, aktiviert werden. Dieses Prinzip der ischämischen Postkonditionierung (IPoC) ist eine Form der verzögerten Reperfusion, wobei die Blutversorgung direkt nach dem Beenden der initialen Ischämie erneut und wiederholt abgeklemmt wird. Die Wirksamkeit dieses Therapieansatzes wurde bereits in verschiedenen Geweben bei unterschiedlichen Tierarten nachgewiesen.

Ziel der vorliegenden Arbeit war es, den Einfluss der pharmakologischen Präkonditionierung (PPC) und der IPoC auf I/R im Dünndarm des Pferdes zu bestimmen. Zu diesem Zweck wurden zwei randomisierte, kontrollierte, experimentelle in vivo Studien durchgeführt. Für beide Studien wurde im Rahmen eines experimentellen Modells bei Pferden in Allgemeinanästhesie eine 90%ige segmentale Jejunumischämie induziert. In der ersten Studie zur Bestimmung der PPC wurden die Pferde entweder mit Xylazin (n=5) oder Lidocain (n=5) präkonditioniert. Eine historische, unbehandelte Kontrollgruppe (n=5) wurde als Vergleichsgruppe verwendet. Für die zweite Studie zur Untersuchung der IPoC, wurde bei der Testgruppe (n=7) eine verzögerte Reperfusion durch wiederholte Abklemmung der Mesenterialgefäße nach Ischämie herbeigeführt. Im Gegensatz dazu wurde bei der Kontrollgruppe die Reperfusion des Jejunums ohne weitere Maßnahmen eingeleitet. Intestinaler Blutfluss und Sauerstoffsättigung wurden in beiden Studien mittels Laser Doppler Flussmessung und Weißlicht Spektrophotometrie gemessen. Darüber hinaus wurden Dünndarmgewebeproben für histologische, immunhistochemische und biochemische Analysen entnommen. Der Vergleich zwischen den Gruppen und Zeitpunkten wurde mittels zweifacher ANOVA und entsprechender post-hoc Tests durchgeführt ($p < 0.05$). Für ordinale und nicht normal verteilte Daten wurden Mann-

Whitney oder Kruskal-Wallis Tests für den Gruppenvergleich sowie Friedman Tests für den Vergleich der Zeitpunkte innerhalb der Gruppen verwendet.

In der ersten Studie (Manuskript 1) ergab PPC mittels Lidocain und Xylazin keine Besserung der durch I/R ausgelösten histomorphologischen Mukosaschädigung. Die Xylazin Therapie führte jedoch zu einer erniedrigten Apoptoserate und einer niedrigeren Anzahl an Entzündungszellen in der Mukosa und Serosa. Die Lidocain Therapie hatte keinen Einfluss auf diese Variablen.

In der IPoC Studie (Manuskript 2 und 3) wurde bei jedem Abklemmungszyklus die Mikroperfusion signifikant verringert. Im Gegensatz dazu wurde die Sauerstoffsättigung lediglich beim ersten Abklemmungszyklus signifikant herabgesetzt. Das Mesenterium einschließlich der dazu gehörenden Gefäße zeigte keine vermehrte Schädigung im Vergleich zur Kontrollgruppe. Die Postkonditionierung bewirkte eine verringerte epitheliale Ablösung und Apoptoserate, sowie eine geringere parazelluläre Permeabilität der Mukosa nach Reperfusion im Vergleich zur Kontrollgruppe. Der Großteil der darüber hinaus getesteten Variablen Histomorphometrie, Zelltod, Entzündung, oxidativer Stress, und 'heat shock response' waren signifikant durch das Ischämie-Modell verändert. Keiner dieser Effekte der I/R wurde allerdings durch die IPoC verringert.

In einem vierten Manuskript wurde darüber hinaus die 'hypoxia inducible factor' (HIF) Antwort im Ischämiemodell sowie der Einfluss von IPoC beschrieben. Nach Reperfusion war die mukosale HIF-1α Immunreaktivität signifikant höher im Vergleich zur Prä-Ischämie. Die HIF-2α Immunreaktivität veränderte sich nicht während Reperfusion und Ischämie. Die Ergebnisse lassen vermuten, dass vorrangig der Transkriptionsfaktor HIF-1α und nicht HIF-2α eine Rolle bei der intestinalen Antwort auf Ischämie spielt. IPoC hatte keinen Einfluss auf das Immunreaktivitätsmuster der beiden Faktoren.

Aufgrund der mit Xylazin PPC einhergehenden Reduktion der apoptotischen und entzündlichen Zellen, kann davon ausgegangen werden, dass Xylazin einen positiven Effekt auf intestinale I/R hat. Dieses Ergebnis unterstützt die Anwendung von Xylazin bei sedativer Analgesie und bei Anästhesieprotokollen bei Pferden mit strangulierenden Dünndarmläsionen. IPoC war zuverlässig und sicher durchzuführen und die Ergebnisse suggerieren einen protektiven Effekt auf I/R assoziierte Beeinträchtigungen der Dünndarmmukosa. Mögliche Wirkungsmechanismen wie das oxidative Stress-Niveau, HIF und 'heat shock response' wurden untersucht, jedoch nicht von IPoC beeinflusst. Das Konzept der IPoC stellt eine Therapieoption mit Potenzial für den Kolikpatienten dar. Nichtsdestotrotz bedürfen der Wirkungsmechanismus und die langfristigen Auswirkungen weiterer Untersuchungen bevor IPOC bei klinischen Fällen zum Einsatz kommen kann.

3. Introduction

3.1. Small intestinal strangulation in horses

3.1.1. Incidence

Colic is a major cause of mortality in horses, representing the single most common cause of death (1). The incidence of colic in different populations of horses has been reported to lie between 3.5 to 10.6 colic episodes per 100 horses per year (2). Of the horses treated for colic in veterinary hospitals, 25% to 64% are affected with small intestinal disease (3-6). The majority of these cases (58% to 85%) are caused by strangulating lesions with concurrent intestinal ischaemia (4-7). The most common strangulating small intestinal lesions in horses are pedunculated lipomas, epiploic foramen entrapment, volvulus and intussusception (3, 8-10).

3.1.2. Pathogenesis

Small intestinal strangulation results in the obstruction of the lumen and the intestinal blood supply. These obstructions can be classified as haemorrhagic or ischaemic strangulating obstructions (11, 12). The first occurs when the veins are occluded more than the arteries, resulting in severe oedema and haemorrhage, also known as warm or low-flow ischaemia (11-14). In contrast, ischaemic strangulating obstructions evoke the complete occlusion of both arterial and venous blood supply, resulting in a pale appearance and rapid tissue degeneration (11, 12, 15, 16). This type of obstruction is also known as cold or no-flow ischaemia.

Intestinal injury occurs as a result of a reduction in oxygen supply. Small intestinal mucosa is known to be very susceptible to ischaemic injury due to its high energy demand and the hypoxic state of the villus tip even under normal conditions (17, 18). On a cellular level, the anaerobic metabolism increases and lactate accumulates, causing a decrease in ATP level and intracellular pH. Ion transport mechanisms become dysfunctional, resulting in calcium overload, cell swelling with subsequent rupture, and cell death by necrotic, necroptotic, apoptotic, and autophagic mechanisms (19). On a histopathological level, this results in the separation of the enterocytes from the lamina propria, inflammatory infiltration, apoptosis and cell necrosis (13, 20). Additionally, seromuscular injury may develop with mesothelial cell loss, leucocytic infiltration and oedema (21). Furthermore, in case of haemorrhagic strangulating obstructions, the resulting haemorrhage may disrupt the tissue architecture (22).

After resolution of the strangulating obstruction, intestinal tissue damage may continue due to reperfusion injury (23, 24). After reestablishment of the blood supply, xanthine oxidase rapidly degrades hypoxanthine thereby producing reactive oxygen species (25). These cause oxidative tissue damage and trigger the arachidonic acid metabolism to generate neutrophil chemo-attractants (26, 27). Even though inflammatory infiltration is considered a part of normal tissue repair, neutrophils can exacerbate tissue injury, and their infiltration during this phase likely contributes to the occurrence of severe post-operative complications such as adhesions and paralytic ileus (12, 28-31). It has been suggested that no-flow ischaemia induces maximal injury during the ischaemic phase (12, 24, 32). Contrarily, experimental studies implementing low flow ischaemia models have demonstrated the occurrence of reperfusion injury in the equine small intestine (14, 32). The significance of reperfusion injury and its contribution to morbidity in clinical cases of strangulating obstruction remains a point of controversy.

3.1.3. Assessment of intestinal viability

Strangulating intestinal obstructions are generally treated by manual resolution of the lesion through a ventral midline laparotomy under general anaesthesia (11, 12). After resolution of the strangulation, the assessment of intestinal viability is of great importance to determine the necessity of small intestinal resection and for determining the prognosis. Colour, wall thickness, presence of peristalsis, and palpable mesenteric arterial pulsation can be used for clinical assessment of the intestine (33). However, changes in colour due to intramural haemorrhage and oedema can be misleading, and it was reported that clinical assessment was only 54% accurate in predicting viability (34). Several ancillary diagnostic methods for the assessment of intestinal lesions have been reviewed, including surface oximetry, Doppler ultrasonography and fluorescein dye (12, 35). However, these methods have not been proven reliable for all types of lesions and clinical application is limited (34). Histology is considered to be the gold standard for determining viability (36, 37). Nevertheless, it is not possible to perform this intra-operatively due to time constraints. Consequently, the clinical assessment remains the most important factor for decision making, even though the crucial factors for and against resection remain a point of discussion among surgeons (12).

3.1.4. Small intestinal resection – prognosis and limitations

If the intestine is judged to be non-viable, small intestinal resection followed by intestinal anastomosis needs to be performed. Survival rates after intestinal resection have increased in the past decades compared to earlier studies (38). Currently, around 80% of the horses survive until discharge, yet a trend towards lower survival rates is found after resection of more than 2 m of intestine (8, 39-41). Adhesions, post-operative ileus and endotoxaemia are common causes of nonsurvival after surgery for small intestinal strangulating obstructions (12). Horses that require small intestinal resection have a poorer short-term survival than horses that do not require resection (42, 43). It must also be noted that in some cases the complete resection of the affected segment may not be possible due to anatomic restrictions, for example in lesions that involve the duodenum or ileum (44). Furthermore, resecting of more than 60 - 75% of the total intestinal length may cause short bowel syndrome (11, 45, 46). Determining the exact site of resection can be precarious, as distension at the periphery of a strangulating lesion can induce injury that is difficult to detect, and resection margins may not be as healthy as would be expected based on the clinical judgement (16, 47). This is of significance, as it has been shown that leaving nonviable small intestine in situ is associated with progressive ischaemic injury, a high rate of early repeat celiotomy and low survival rates (42, 48). Consequently, all these factors need to be considered and complicate the decision making in the surgical treatment of small intestinal strangulating lesions.

3.1.5. Adjunctive treatment strategies

As mentioned in the previous section, small intestinal resection cannot serve as the solution for all cases of strangulating obstructions. Moreover, assessment of intestinal viability has not been proven to be highly reliable, and grossly unaltered intestinal tissue may already have undergone irreversible damage only apparent at histological level. Therefore, alternative treatment strategies are necessary to ameliorate ischaemia reperfusion injury of the intestine during colic surgery. Although the clinical significance of reperfusion injury is inconclusive at this time, many pharmacological substances have been tested for their ability to attenuate oxidative damage after intestinal ischaemia. Experimental trials in equine small intestinal ischaemia models have investigated the administration of DMSO, Allopurinol, intraluminal oxygen and 21-Aminosteroid without detecting a reduction in mucosal injury (32, 49). In contrast, the local application of customized solutions containing combinations of different substances such as allopurinol, deferoxamine and adenosine did ameliorate mucosal and microvascular injury (50, 51). Superoxide dismutase, lidocaine, platelet-activating factor antagonist, high-molecular-weight dextrans, manganese chloride, and acetylcysteine have also been tested in experimental trials, with variable success (27, 52-55). Clinical trials are lacking, and except for the use of systemic lidocaine, these therapies have not found acceptance and implementation in clinical practice.

3.2. Preconditioning

As in veterinary medicine, ischaemic injury of different organs and tissues has a significant impact in human medicine. Especially ischaemic heart diseases cost many lives each year (56). They represent a major drive for the development of new treatment strategies to ameliorate myocardial ischaemia reperfusion injury. This is how the concept of preconditioning came into life. This phenomenon abides by the principle of hormesis which refers to the adaptive cellular responses after exposure to low doses of a noxious stimulus, increasing the tolerance of the cell or tissue to higher levels of a noxious stimulus (57).

3.2.1. Ischaemic preconditioning

Ischaemic or mechanical preconditioning was first discovered in 1986 by Murry et al. (58), who demonstrated that myocardial infarction in dogs was reduced by 75% when four cycles of 5 min coronary artery occlusion preceded 40 min of coronary ischaemia. Following this discovery, the phenomenon was extensively investigated in rodent, rabbit and canine models of myocardial ischaemia, demonstrating reduced infarct size and apoptosis rate, decreased neutrophil accumulation, preserved vascular endothelial function and attenuation of the incidence and severity of post-ischaemic arrhythmias (59-63). This led to the implementation of ischaemic preconditioning by aortic clamping in human patients subjected to coronary artery bypass surgery. Reported positive effects were reductions in postoperative troponin release, improvements in the cardiac index, and a reduction in the need for postoperative inotropic support (64-66). Contrarily, other studies could not detect a positive effect on oxygen saturation, arterial pH, blood lactate, creatinine kinase and troponin release (67, 68).

The increasing popularity of IPC did not remain unnoticed in other medical fields; hence this concept was also adapted to other organs. For example, the cytoprotective effects have been demonstrated in the liver in several studies using a rat model (69, 70), and IPC was found to be an effective treatment against hepatic ischaemia in human patients undergoing hemihepatectomy (71).

In the field of small intestinal ischaemia, various experimental studies have been performed. The most commonly used experimental model is the occlusion of the cranial mesenteric artery (CMA) in rats, with significant variations in the time frame of the experiment. The duration of the main ischaemic event usually varied between 30 to 90 minutes, and the preconditioning ischaemic bouts ranged between 2 minutes and 1 hour, with 5 or 10 minutes being most commonly reported (72-78). Some authors who compared different IPC regimes demonstrated better protection with cycles of a shorter duration of 2 to 10 minutes (79, 80). It has also been shown that repeated episodes of ischaemia induce a better protective effect than a single ischaemic period (81). Another point of variation is the reperfusion time between preconditioning and main ischaemic episode, with a range between 5 minutes and 24 hours (72-78, 82).

These experimental studies have investigated many different aspects of intestinal ischaemia reperfusion injury. IPC was found to reduce the histomorphological changes in the intestinal mucosa (76, 78, 79, 83-87) and to induce less intestinal oedema with lower wet-to-dry ratios (77, 85). Lower apoptosis rates were reported, based on immunohistochemical staining for M30 (75, 76) or by Terminal deoxynucleotidyl transferase dUTP Nick-End Labeling (TUNEL) (72, 88). IPC was also associated with lower myeloperoxidase (MPO) activity as a marker for inflammation (76-78).

Evaluating oxidative stress variables, IPC reduced the generation of reactive oxygen species (88), and biochemical analysis of blood serum revealed decreased serum lactic dehydrogenase and lactate levels following IPC (83, 85, 86, 89). The intestinal tissue exhibited lower malondialdehyde levels and higher superoxide dismutase activity (72, 76-78). Furthermore, a lower percentage of xanthine dehydrogenase to xanthine oxidase conversion, uric acid concentration, and reduced glutathione were found in preconditioned rats (90). Looking at the effect on the barrier function of the mucosa, IPC ameliorated intestinal hyperpermeability (84) and prevented I/R-induced bacterial translocation (87). Other functional parameters that were improved by IPC include the transit of intestinal content (78), intestinal microvascular perfusion and tissue oxygenation (86), and reperfusion-induced hypotension (85). A study investigating IPC in a pig model with occlusion of the CMA found similar results to those reported in the rat model (73).

Most studies investigated the short-term effects of IPC with reperfusion times limited to 30 to 120 minutes, with only few authors applying a longer duration of reperfusion. At 24 hours, IPC improved the mucosal perfusion and decreased the leukocyte-endothelial interactions, as shown by intravital fluorescence microscopy (91), and a similar positive effect on MPO levels and transit of intestinal content compared to the effect after 6 hours was shown (78). The effect of IPC on histomorphology at this time point was variable, with one group reporting a significant effect of IPC (91), while another could not confirm this (78).

Because IPC can be applied prior to organ transplantation, this treatment strategy has also been used in experimental models for small intestinal grafting with segments of jejunum. In rats, IPC decreased the mucosal histological damage and LDH, AST and ALT levels (92, 93). Other reported positive effects were lower MPO levels (93), a lower apoptotic index, and a lesser degree of epithelial basement membrane disruption, as shown by transmission electron microscopy (94). An experimental study in pigs found higher levels of GSH and SOD as well as decreased oxygen free radicals (95). The same research group reported similar results when it performed the same experiment in dogs (96).

One experimental study in horses found that IPC prevented the progression of histological injury during reperfusion, yet IPC was also associated with increased infiltration of inflammatory cells (97). To the author's knowledge, there are so far no reports of the implementation of intestinal IPC in clinical trials in any species.

3.2.2. Pharmacological preconditioning

Preconditioning with pharmacological agents can also ameliorate ischaemic injury. After the discovery of ischaemic preconditioning, a substantial number of studies were performed that followed the concept of pharmacological preconditioning (PPC). As with IPC, most studies were undertaken in experimental myocardial ischaemia models, and a wide range in pharmacological agents have been shown to induce intrinsic protective mechanisms against ischaemia and reperfusion injury (98, 99). The pharmacological substances that have been tested can be divided into two categories. Firstly, specific triggers and signalling molecules have been investigated to determine the mechanisms behind IPC. Furthermore, drugs that are used in clinical practice have been tested for their ability to mimic the effect of and possibly replace IPC.

The most commonly reported effects of intestinal IPC were also demonstrated after PPC. A variety of pharmacological substances were shown to reduce histomorphological injury, apoptosis, and biomarkers for oxidative stress and inflammation (76, 100-102). Examples of triggers or downstream signalling molecules tested for ameliorating intestinal injury are adenosine (76, 101), calcitonin gene-related peptide (100) and erythropoietin (103). PPC with Vitamin C also attenuated intestinal injury (104). Furthermore, in an attempt to elucidate how the protective effect of IPC is mediated, substances that specifically inhibit possible target receptors have been extensively investigated. This topic will be reviewed in more detail in the section on the mechanism of action (chapter 3.5).

More relevant for direct translation to clinical cases are studies investigating the PPC effect of drugs used in clinical practice. Volatile anaesthetics such as isoflurane and sevoflurane exhibit a dose-dependent preconditioning effect against IR-induced renal and intestinal injury (101, 105). Pretreatment with morphine prior to ischaemia and reperfusion mimicked the protection induced by intestinal IPC (77). N-acetylcysteine preconditioning in pigs undergoing small intestinal transplantation reduced the systemic levels of inflammatory markers (106). Several studies have reported the PPC effect of the highly selective α2-adrenergic receptor agonist dexmedetomidine on intestinal injury in rabbits and rats (102, 107). Moreover, this protective effect could also be demonstrated in an experimental model of equine small intestinal strangulation (97, 108). Of the above mentioned drugs only the inhalation anaesthetics are routinely used in the anaesthetic management of horses. The administration of dexmedetomidine has also been proven safe and effective in horses (109); however, there are no commercially available formulations that are registered for horses. Xylazine and lidocaine, both routinely used in the management of small intestinal colic (110), have not been investigated for their ability to elicit PPC.

3.3. Postconditioning

3.3.1. Ischaemic postconditioning

Due to the unpredictable nature of most ischaemic events, the concept of preconditioning is of limited practicability as treatment for patients with acute ischaemic disease. Almost 20 years after the discovery of preconditioning, the principle of ischaemic postconditioning (IPoC) was introduced. This first report of IPoC demonstrated that gradual and controlled reperfusion was more effective than abrupt elimination of the vascular occlusion in salvaging the ischaemic myocardium in dogs (111). This builds on the hypothesis that the protective mechanisms exerted by preconditioning may be activated after the blood supply has been reinstated (112). Ischaemic postconditioning is defined as delayed reperfusion by the repeated re-occlusion of the relevant blood vessels directly after an ischaemic event (99, 111).

As with IPC, most studies were performed in the field of cardiology. Experimental trials investigating myocardial ischaemia in rats subjected to IPoC found a decrease in the size of myocardial infarcts and less extensive oedema, reduced occurrence of arrhythmias, lower oxidative stress levels, reduced MPO activity, and improved ion pump function (111, 113-115). This has led to the application of IPoC in human patients with acute myocardial infarction, where postconditioning can be applied after thrombolysis by reocclusion of the coronary artery with an intravascular balloon catheter (116, 117). A meta-analysis of clinical trials has identified beneficial effects of this treatment in some of the tested variables, reporting improvement in the myocardial salvage index and decreased myocardial oedema, yet without affecting final infarct size, left ventricular volume or microvascular obstruction (118).

A protective effect of IPoC has also been reported in experimental ischaemia of liver (119), kidney (120), brain (121), lung (122), spinal cord (123), and testis (124). Furthermore, a large set of experimental trials in the rat CMA model for small intestinal ischaemia have shown many beneficial effects in rats subjected to IPoC (72, 125-133). Comparable to the situation with IPC, it is a topic of discussion whether the efficacy of IPoC is primarily due to the number of cycles, the duration of each cycle, or the total duration of the IPoC algorithm. As with intestinal IPC, shorter and more frequent cycles of 5 - 10 seconds seem to confer better intestinal protection than re-occlusion cycles of longer duration (130, 131, 134). On the other hand, one study found no difference between 2 cycles of 2 minutes and 4 cycles of 30 secs (135). Regarding the timing of IPoC, it seems to be essential that it is initiated immediately after abolishment of ischaemia, since one study reported that the protective effects of IPoC were lost when it was first performed after 3 minutes (126).

Similar to the results of the intestinal IPC studies, IPoC was found to reduce histomorphological injury of the mucosa (72, 125-133), intestinal oedema (126, 132), and the amount of TUNEL positive apoptotic cells (72, 127-129). Furthermore, IPoC decreased the expression of cleaved caspase-3 and -9 (127, 128). Other signs of apoptosis and cell death such as DNA ladder formation after electrophoresis (72) and serum levels of intestinal-type fatty acid-binding protein (127) were also reduced by IPoC.

Expression of biomarkers for oxidative stress was significantly lower in the groups subjected to IPoC. This was reflected by lower plasma and tissue levels of MDA (72, 126, 128, 130), lactate (128, 132), LDH (127, 131), creatine kinase (CK) (130, 131), and diamine oxidase (DAO) (128). Furthermore, IPoC increased the levels of superoxide dismutase (SOD) (128) and caused less reduction in the concentration of the free thiol groups (131).

Inflammatory signs were found to be lower in the IPoC groups, reflected by lower plasma and tissue MPO levels (72, 126, 136). Moreover, plasma concentrations of tumour necrosis factor (TNF)-α and interleukin (IL)-6 were lower after IPoC (126, 131). Evaluating the mucosal barrier function after IPoC, one study reported reduced bacterial translocation and higher values for mean arterial pressure (137). Furthermore, IPoC has been shown to decrease the claudin-2 immunoreactivity in epithelial cells after ischaemia (137).

Only little research has been done in other animal models. Implementation of IPoC in a CMA occlusion model in mice resulted in decreased histomorphological injury and lower serum levels of intestinal-type fatty acid-binding protein, TNF-α and IL-6 (138, 139). One study that investigated segmental jejunal ischaemia in rabbits could not detect an influence of IPoC on the tested variables of mucosal histomorphology and intestinal wet-to-dry ratio (140). In a pig model for small bowel transplantation, IPoC reduced MDA concentration and increased glutathione and SOD levels (141). To the author's knowledge, no studies on the effect of IPoC have so far been performed in horses. Furthermore, no clinical reports of intestinal IPoC are available.

3.3.2. Pharmacological postconditioning

Comparable to PPC, pharmacological substances have also been found to mimic the effects of ischaemic conditioning when administered immediately after the ischaemic event. Most studies investigating pharmacological postconditioning (PPoC), have focused on mimicking or abolishing the effects of IPoC by stimulation or inhibition of certain triggers and receptors, to find out more about its mode of action. Many drugs that have shown a protective effect in PPC have also been tested for their PPoC ability, among them several anaesthetics that may be of clinical relevance in the horse. Post-ischaemic administration of sevoflurane has been shown to ameliorate mucosal injury and inflammation in pigs and rats (101, 142). PPoC with propofol alleviated pathological changes in intestines and lung, and decreased apoptosis and oxidative stress levels (143). One study that investigated dexmedetomidine PPC in horses also found decreased epithelial injury scores following dexmedetomidine PPoC (108).

An extensive discussion of all substances that have been investigated as PPoC mediator goes beyond the scope of this thesis and can be found in published reviews on this topic (98, 99, 144). Moreover, it must be noted that drugs eliciting a protective effect during reperfusion do not necessarily exert this protection through the mechanism of postconditioning in the sense of hormesis. Nonetheless, the increasing popularity of postconditioning has led to the widespread adaptation of this term for the administration of drugs following ischaemia.

3.4. Remote conditioning

Another treatment strategy that has been discovered in relation to ischaemic conditioning is remote conditioning (RC). This describes the phenomenon that the protective effects of IPC and IPoC are not limited to the organ directly exposed to the bouts of conditioning ischaemia (99). Such protection in organs distant to those that are preconditioned enables the initiation of cell survival programmes in tissues that cannot be preconditioned directly in clinical situations. Remote conditioning has been shown to elicit a protective effect when performed prior to the main ischaemic event (remote preconditioning)(145), or directly after ischaemia (remote postconditioning) (146). This concept has been explored in different organs, mainly applying upper or lower limb ischaemia with a tourniquet as remote conditioning stimulus (145, 147-149). Alternatively, intraoperative occlusion of the infrarenal aorta, the renal artery or the hepatic pedicle have been performed (146, 150, 151). Experimental studies have reported attenuated ischaemia reperfusion injury following remote conditioning in different organs including the heart (146), the brain (147), the spinal cord (148), the kidney (151), and the small intestine (149, 150).

Remote conditioning has been applied to clinical cases, mainly human patients undergoing cardiac or renal surgey, or suffering from acute cerebral infarction (152-155). Resulting clinical trials have reported variable beneficial effects (152-155). In clinical cases of kidney transplantation, remote preconditioning was feasible and safe, yet no benefit in terms of the clinical outcome was observed (156). Remote postconditioning after acute cerebral infarction was associated with improvement in some of the tested variables, including stroke scores and several biomarkers (157). In experimental intestinal ischaemia RC significantly reduced histological damage, inflammation and oxidative stress in the rat CMA model (158, 159). Lower limb ischaemia can also cause remote injury to the gastrointestinal system, and remote postconditioning can have a protective effect on this type of injury, with reduced histological damage and increased intestinal blood flow (150) as well as reduced expression of biomarkers for inflammation and oxidative stress (149). An experimental study looking at small intestinal anastomosis healing could not detect a beneficial effect of remote preconditioning (160). There are no reports on the application of RC in clinical patients with intestinal ischaemia.

3.5. Conditioning – the mechanism of action

Many studies in different tissues and experimental models have shown a protective effect of pre-, post- or remote conditioning. Similarly, a great amount of research has been dedicated to find the protective mechanism behind this phenomenon. Even though there may be differences between the different strategies, tissues and species, many of the identified triggers and pathways seem to play a role in all of them. It has been suggested that these pathways are activated during early reperfusion in both IPC and IPoC, possibly explaining the similar mechanism of action despite the difference in timing (112). The protective effects can be divided into an early phase of protection which induces the activation of pre-existing effectors, and a late phase of protection mediated by the upregulation of cytoprotective proteins (Fig.1) (99, 147, 161, 162).

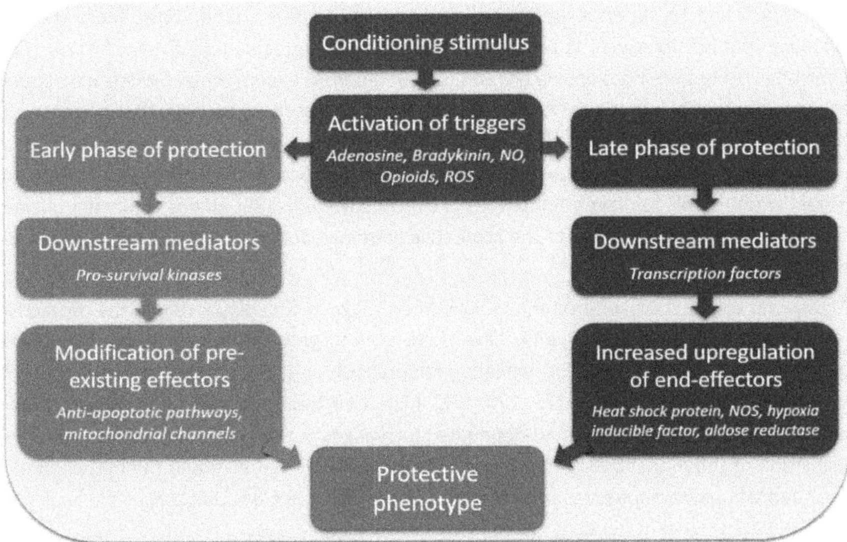

Figure 1: Diagram illustrating the proposed mechanism of action of conditioning (99, 147, 161, 162).

Using models of acute myocardial and intestinal ischaemia it has been shown that the protective effects of pre- and postconditioning are mediated by the activation of adenosine (76, 84, 163-165), bradykinin (166, 167), and opioid receptors (77, 168-170). The next step in the conditioning signalling cascade is the activation of pro-survival kinases such as PI3K/Akt and ERK-1/2, (112, 171, 172). With regard to intestinal postconditioning, the activation of Akt (133, 139), Nrf2 (133) and the JAK/STAT pathway (136) have been identified. These pro-survival pathways may initiate the expression of specific micro-RNAs (miR) and circular RNAs for subsequent regulation of protein expression (138). Several studies have found increased expression of miR-21 in response to IPC and IPoC (129, 172, 173). Another possible signalling molecule is nitric oxide. There are several studies that detected an increase in the synthesis of nitric oxide after ischaemic conditioning, and found that inhibition of nitric oxide synthesis abolished the protective effect of IPC (87, 89, 93).

A potential signalling protein that has received a lot of attention in the last few years is hypoxia inducible factor 1-alpha (HIF-1α). HIF-1α mediates many effects of hypoxia by acting as transcription factor (174, 175). HIF-dependent regulation of claudin-1 plays an important role in maintenance of intestinal epithelial tight junction integrity (176). Moreover, it has been shown that HIF-1α expression increases in ischaemic intestinal mucosa (177). The expression of the isoform HIF-2α is also increased in different tissues including the intestine under hypoxic conditions (178). However, HIF-2α has so far not been investigated in intestinal ischaemia. It has been suggested that HIF-1α plays a signalling role in the protective mechanism of IPoC. In experimental models of intestinal and myocardial ischaemia, HIF-1α expression was higher in groups subjected to IPoC compared to the untreated control groups, and was accompanied by less tissue damage (129, 179, 180). Remote conditioning and PPoC have also found to be associated with increased HIF-1α levels (154, 158). There is some evidence that HIF-1α exerts its protective effect through upregulation of miR-21 (129, 180). Contrarily, other investigations on IPC and IPoC in different experimental models have found an association between HIF-1α levels and the extent of tissue injury (181-183). In horses, it was found that manipulated intestinal tissue exhibited lower HIF-1α levels compared to control tissue (184). It has been suggested that the duration and severity of the I/R insult dictate whether HIF-1α plays a deleterious or a protective role (185). Hence, it remains unclear if HIF-1α represents a marker for the protective response, for the degree of I/R injury, or for both.

A great variety of downstream targets have been suggested to play a role in the protective mechanism of conditioning (99, 144). One of the main targets is the attenuation of apoptosis by modulating the expression of regulating factors such as *BCL-2* protein, as shown in both myocardial and intestinal IPoC (75, 170, 172). Increased expression of LC3 II/I, Beclin-1, and p62 was shown to mediate an IPoC-dependent increase in autophagy (133). Furthermore, the regulation of the mitochondrial permeability transition pores (mPTP) and the mitochondrial K_{ATP} channels appears to represent a common end effector (85, 88, 186-188).

The upregulation of protective proteins has also been suggested to be of importance, especially in the late phase of protection (147). An example of such proteins are the heat shock proteins (HSP). HSP function as molecular chaperones and are upregulated in response to a variety of noxious stimuli (189). Especially the HSP-70 family has been shown to play a protective role in the intestine, with upregulation after intestinal I/R in different animal models (190, 191), and significantly less intestinal necrosis after zinc mediated induction of this protein (192). Upregulation of HSP-70 has been reported after RC and IPC in the brain, spinal cord and heart, and has been linked to miR mediated signalling (147, 148, 173). Heme-Oxygenase-1 also belongs to the HSP-family. It is the equivalent of inducible HSP-32 (189) and exerts a cytoprotective effect through the reduction of oxidative stress and inflammation (193). Several studies have identified heme-oxygenase-1 as an important factor in IPC, RC and IPoC mediated protection (82, 91, 104, 139). Other proteins that have been suggested as effector of ischaemic conditioning are aldose reductase (128) and calcitonin gene-related peptide (100).

Several studies have evaluated the possible mechanism behind PPC and PPoC and report that the direct activation of pro-survival kinases mediates the effect of dexmedetomidine and sevoflurane (101, 194). It has also been suggested that dexmedetomidine preconditioning may trigger an ischaemic event mediated by alpha-2 adrenergic stimulation and consecutive vasoconstriction, producing an effect similar to IPC (195, 196).

Apart from the above-mentioned mediators of IPC and IPoC protection, IPoC may have an additional mode of action. It has been hypothesised that this delayed reperfusion may also slow down the washout of protective factors such as adenosine or bradykinin (99). Furthermore, it has been shown that IPoC can delay the restoration of acidosis, and thereby limits sodium and calcium overload and possibly prevents mPTP formation (131, 188).

4. Aims and Objectives

With the need for additional treatments for small intestinal I/R injury in horses, pharmacological preconditioning may represent a feasible strategy during the anaesthetic management of horses with colic. Dexmedetomidine has been shown to elicit a protective effect in horses, yet drugs that are more commonly used in the clinical management of colic in horses have not been evaluated for their preconditioning abilities. Therefore, the aim of the first part of this study was to investigate whether xylazine and lidocaine have a preconditioning effect on equine small intestinal ischaemia. We hypothesised that preconditioning with xylazine or lidocaine would ameliorate I/R injury. The objective was to evaluate the histomorphology and the extent of apoptosis and inflammatory cell infiltration in the intestine after experimental segmental jejunal ischaemia in the horse, and to assess the effect of xylazine and lidocaine administration on these variables.

Ischaemic postconditioning could hold an additional therapeutic potential for the ischaemic intestinal segments that are not reached by preconditioning. Results from experimental laboratory animal models investigating intestinal IPoC are promising; however, there are no reports of this technique in horses, or of comparable clinical approaches in any species. Consequently, the aim of the second part of the study was to determine whether IPoC can ameliorate I/R injury in the equine small intestine. The primary objective was to assess the feasibility of IPoC in the equine jejunum, and to evaluate the effect of this treatment strategy on experimental small intestinal I/R injury. The following hypotheses and secondary objectives were formulated:

1. IPoC is feasible and safe to perform in the equine jejunum.
    - The objective was to measure the intestinal blood flow and tissue oxygen saturation during IPoC with modified haemostatic clamps, and to apply histology to assess the damage to the mesentery and its vessels after clamping.
2. Intestinal mucosal morphology and function is better preserved after IPoC.
    - The objective was to assess histomorphology, nutritional transport, and paracellular permeability of the intestinal mucosal in a group of horses subjected to postconditioning and an untreated control group.
3. IPoC decreases intestinal cell death, inflammation, and oxidative stress.
    - The objective was to compare different intestinal tissue markers for inflammation, cell death and oxidative stress between the groups.
4. IPoC is associated with a more pronounced heat shock and hypoxia inducible factor response.
    - The objective was to assess the intestinal distribution and expression of Heat Shock Protein-70 and hypoxia inducible factors 1α and 2α during equine experimental ischaemia, and compare this response between the groups.

5. Manuscript I

Preconditioning with lidocaine and xylazine in experimental equine jejunal ischaemia

N. Verhaar[1], C. Pfarrer[2], S. Neudeck[1], K. König[1], K. Rohn[3], L. Twele[1], S. Kästner[1,4]

[1] Clinic for Horses, University of Veterinary Medicine Hannover, Germany

[2] Institute for Anatomy, University of Veterinary Medicine Hannover, Germany

[3] Department of Biometry, University of Veterinary Medicine Hannover, Germany

[4] Small Animal Clinic, University of Veterinary Medicine Hannover, Germany

Published in Equine Veterinary Journal (2021) 53 (1): 125-133

doi.org/10.1111/evj.13251

Author contribution

- NV contributed to the study design and execution, performed the microscopic examination, as well as the data analysis and interpretation, and prepared the manuscript.
- CP and SK contributed to the study design as well as the data interpretation.
- SN, KK and LT contributed to the study design and its execution.
- KR was involved in the data analysis.
- All authors edited or contributed to the manuscript.

Summary

Background: Pharmacological preconditioning of dexmedetomidine on small intestinal ischaemia/reperfusion (I/R) injury has been reported in different animal models including horses.

Objectives: The objective was to assess if xylazine and lidocaine have a preconditioning effect in an experimental model of equine jejunal ischaemia.

Study design: Terminal in vivo experiment.

Methods: Ten horses under general anaesthesia were either preconditioned with xylazine (group X; n=5) or lidocaine (group L; n=5). A historical untreated control group (group C; n=5) was used for comparison. An established experimental model of equine jejunal ischaemia was applied, and intestinal samples were taken pre-ischaemia, after ischaemia and following reperfusion. Histomorphological examination was performed based on a modified Chiu score. Immunohistochemical staining for cleaved-caspase-3, TUNEL and calprotectin were performed, and positive cell counts were expressed in cells/mm^2.

Results: There was no progression of histomorphological mucosal injury from ischaemia to reperfusion, and there were no differences in histomorphology between the groups. After ischaemia, group X had significantly less caspase positive cells compared to the control group (p=0.01). Group X also exhibited significantly lower calprotectin positive cell counts in the mucosa and serosa than the control group after reperfusion (p=0.02 and 0.05, respectively). All groups showed an increase in caspase and calprotectin positive cells during reperfusion (p<0.05). TUNEL positive cells increased during ischaemia, followed by a decrease after reperfusion (p<0.05).

Main limitations: The small sample size and the use of a historical control group. Preconditioning effects of the tested drugs may be masked by the protective effects of isoflurane in the anaesthetic protocol.

Conclusions: Preconditioning with lidocaine did not have any effect on the tested variables. The lower cell counts of caspase and calprotectin positive cells in group X may indicate a beneficial effect of xylazine on I/R injury. Due to the absence of a concurrent reduction of histomorphological injury, the clinical significance remains uncertain.

Introduction

Small intestinal strangulation with concurrent ischaemia/reperfusion (I/R) injury is a major cause of mortality in horses [1]. An increasingly popular mechanism for the treatment of ischaemic lesions in human medicine is ischaemic preconditioning (IPC) [2]. This refers to the activation of intrinsic cell survival programs after exposure to mild ischaemic stimuli or pharmacologic agents, and several studies have demonstrated the beneficial effect of IPC on the survival of intestinal tissue [3]. Besides mechanical ischaemic preconditioning, many different pharmacological agents like volatile anaesthetics and alpha-2-agonists, have been shown to activate these protective cell responses [2]. Some authors have reported the pharmacological preconditioning (PPC) effect of the alpha-2-agonist dexmedetomidine on intestinal injury in rabbits and rats [4; 5]. Moreover, a protective effect of dexmedetomidine was identified in an experimental model of equine small intestinal strangulation [6]. This beneficial effect may be due to its anti-inflammatory and anti-apoptotic properties [4]. To the authors' knowledge there are no reports on a PPC effect of xylazine, a more commonly used alpha-2-agonist in horses.

Lidocaine is the most commonly used prokinetic drug in the peri-operative management of horses undergoing colic surgery [7]. In experimental models it has been shown to have a beneficial effect on the intestine after ischaemia and reperfusion (I/R), by decreasing intestinal oedema [8], decreasing COX-2 expression in intestinal mucosa [9], and by limiting the increased gut wall permeability compared to flunixin–meglumine administration alone [10]. In a more recent experimental study, the horses treated with lidocaine did not show a consistent decrease in intestinal neutrophil infiltration compared to the untreated horses [11]. Up to date, the exact mechanism of these actions remains unclear. To the authors' knowledge, no studies have been done to explore if there is a preconditioning effect of lidocaine in horses.

The aim of this study was to investigate whether xylazine and lidocaine, which are routinely used in the management of small intestinal colic, have a preconditioning effect on equine jejunal ischaemia. The objective was to describe histomorphology, apoptosis and inflammatory cell count in the intestinal tissue undergoing experimental ischaemia, and to compare these results between different treatment groups. The authors hypothesize that preconditioning with xylazine or lidocaine will ameliorate I/R injury. Identifying a preconditioning effect of either pharmacologic agent would support its use in sedation protocols and anaesthetic regimens for horses with colic.

Material and Methods

Animals

The study was reviewed by the Ethics Committee for Animal Experiments of Lower Saxony, Germany, and approved according to the German Animal Welfare Act. For this terminal in vivo experiment, 10 adult warmblood horses were randomly assigned to a lidocaine group (group L; n=5) or a xylazine (group X; n =5). Group L comprised of 3 mares, 1 gelding and 1 stallion, with an age range of 9 to 19 years (12 ± 4 years, mean ± standard deviation) and the weight ranging between 540 and 619 kg (573 ± 31 kg). Group X comprised of 4 mares and 1 stallion, with an age range of 4 to 21 years (14 ± 8 years), and the weight between 520 and 705 kg (577 ± 76 kg). A historical control group consisting of five warmblood horses, with an age range of 2–14 years (5.4 ± 4.9 years) and the weight between 464 and 610 kg (544 ± 53 kg) was used to limit the amount of horses needed. This control group was taken from a previous study performed by this research group evaluating the preconditioning effect of dexmedetomidine

[6], using the same experimental model, anaesthetic regime and sample preparation as the current study. The horses were acquired by the equine hospital for educational purposes in the anatomy department of the university, and they were elected for euthanasia due to problems unrelated to the gastrointestinal tract, such as orthopaedic disease. All horses were systemically healthy without any signs of gastrointestinal disorders. At least two weeks prior to surgery, the horses were stabled at the facilities of the equine clinic and no medication was administered during this time. The horses had free access to hay and water and were hand walked daily. Six hours before surgery feed but not water was withheld.

Anaesthetic protocol and monitoring

Before the procedure, a 12-gauge Teflon catheter (Intraflon[1a]) was placed in the left jugular vein. In the control group (group C; n=5), anaesthesia was induced without prior sedation. The horses were infused with 5% guaifenesin (My-50 mg/mLl[2b]) until ataxia was apparent. At this point 0.05 mg/kg diazepam (Ziapam 5mg/kg[3c]) and 2.5 mg/kg ketamine (Narketan[4d)]) were administered to induce general anaesthesia. Orotracheal intubation was performed and anaesthesia was maintained with isoflurane (Isofluran CP[2b]) in 100% oxygen. The horses in group L were anaesthetised according to the same protocol, and additionally received a loading dose of 1.3 mg kg BW lidocaine (Lidocain 2%[5e]) over 10 min prior to induction. Subsequently, a continuous rate infusion (CRI) of lidocaine at a rate of 0.05 mg/kg/min was instituted within 5 minutes after induction [12]. Group X, received a loading dose of 1 mg/kg xylazine (Xylavet 20 mg/ml[2b]) over 10 minutes prior to induction of anaesthesia, followed by a CRI of 1 mg/kg/h [13]. In group C, lactated Ringer's solution (Ringer-Laktat EcobagClick[6f]) and dobutamine (Dobutamin-ratiopharm 250mg[7g]) were given at a constant rate of 5 ml/kg/h and 0.5 µg/kg/min, respectively. In group L and X, lactated Ringer's solution was started at 5 ml/kg/h and increased stepwise in increments of 5ml/kg/h to a maximum of 20 ml/kg/h to maintain a mean arterial blood pressure (MAP) above 60 mmHg. This was supplemented by a CRI of dobutamine at a rate of 0.3 µg/kg/min if the initial increase in intravenous fluid rate did not have an effect, and subsequently titrated with increments of 0.3 µg/kg/min. This stepwise approach was continued until the MAP reached the desired level above 60 mmHg. If the MAP rose above 80 mmHg, the rates were decreased in the same manner. During the procedure, cardiovascular and respiratory values were monitored and documented every 10 minutes. Direct arterial blood pressure measurement and arterial and mixed venous blood gas analyses were performed, as well as cardiac output measurement by thermodilution as described previously [14]. The cardiac index (CI) was determined by dividing the cardiac output by the body weight, and the oxygen extraction ratio (OER) was calculated as the ratio of the difference between the arterial and mixed venous blood oxygen content to the arterial blood oxygen content.

Surgical procedure and sample collection

After induction of anaesthesia, the horses were positioned in dorsal recumbency. Sixty minutes after induction of anaesthesia, a routine pre-umbilical midline laparotomy was performed. At 90 minutes, the distal jejunum was exteriorized and a 10-cm intestinal segment located 1 m oral to the jejuno-ileal junction was excised after ligation of the blood vessels and the intestinal lumen (pre-ischaemia (P) sample). Subsequently, ischaemia was induced in a jejunal segment located 2 m oral to the jejunoileal junction by occluding the intestine and mesentery with umbilical tape under monitoring of tissue blood flow and saturation by micro-lightguide spectrophotometry and laser Doppler flowmetry (O2C Oxygen to See[h])[15] until the blood flow was reduced to 10% of the pre ligation measurement. Ninety minutes after initiation of low-flow ischaemia, a 10-cm intestinal segment was excised from the ischaemic area (ischaemia (I) sample). Subsequently, the ligature was released under monitoring with the O2C® to confirm restoration of blood flow. After 30 minutes of reperfusion, an intestinal segment from the previously occluded area was resected (reperfusion (R) sample). After the last sample was taken, the horses were euthanized by intravenous administration of 90 mg/kg pentobarbital (Release 50 mg/ml[i]) without regaining consciousness.

Sample preparation

The intestinal samples were fixed in 4% formaldehyde and embedded in paraffin. Four µm thick sections were cut and the slides were stained routinely with haematoxylin and eosin (H&E) for histomorphological examination. Immunohistochemical staining was performed for cleaved caspase 3 as marker for apoptosis, and for terminal deoxynucleotidyl transferase dUTP nick end labeling (TUNEL) as marker for late-apoptosis and cell necrosis. The staining for cleaved caspase 3 was performed using commercial antibodies (CleavedCaspase-3Asp175 antibody[j]). The complete staining protocol is provided in supplementary item 1. A commercial kit was used for the immunohistochemical staining of TUNEL (ApopTag® Peroxidase In Situ Apoptosis Detection Kit[k]). This was performed according to the manufacturer's instructions. Furthermore, immunohistochemical staining for cytosolic calprotectin was performed using monoclonal mouse anti-human myeloid/histiocyte antigen (clone MAC 387[l]) as described elsewhere [16].

Histomorphological and immunohistochemical examination

The histomorphological and immunohistochemical examination of all the slides including those of the historical control group was performed by the same observer, after being blinded to the sample type and group assignment. This observer (NV) was trained by an experienced histologist (CP). The histomorphological properties of the mucosa were assessed by light microscopy(AXIO Scope.A1[m]) in H&E stained slides in 10 adjoined high-power fields (HPF's) at a 400-fold magnification using a modified Chiu score [17; 18] One slide per time point per horse was assessed. Each field of view was scored individually, and subsequently averaged to make up the final score of each slide. In this modified Chiu score, the villous morphology and the degree of haemorrhage in the tissue were scored separately (Table 1).

TABLE 1: Description of the modified Chiu score with a separated villous and haemorrhage score

Modified Chiu score	*Villi score*	*Haemorrhage score*
0	Normal mucosal villi	None
1	Development of subepithelial (Gruenhagen's) space at the apex of the villus	Dilated capillaries in the lamina propria
2	Extension of the subepithelial space with moderate lifting of the lamina propria	Local haemorrhage in the lamina propria
3	Severe epithelial separation down the villus sides, until halfway down the villus	Diffuse haemorrhage in the lamina propria
4	Denuded villi with the lamina propria exposed	Subepithelial haemorrhage
5	Digestion and disintegration of the lamina propria and ulceration	Massive haemorrhage

The TUNEL- and caspase-3-positive cells in the mucosa were counted in 10 adjoined HPF's per slide. By use of a microscope camera and accompanying software (Axiocam 105 color and Software ZEN 2.3[m]), the exact surface area was determined in mm^2 and the apoptotic cell count was expressed in cells/mm^2. For the calprotectin stain, the number of positive cells in the mucosa were counted in five adjoined HPF's per slide and the count was expressed as cells per mm^2. Additionally, the positive cells within 30 randomly identified submucosal venules were counted. In the submucosa and muscularis, very few positive cells were located outside the vasculature (<1/HPF), hence these layers were not included in the counts. Positive cells in the serosa were counted over the width of 5 HPF's.

Statistical analyses

Prior to commencing the study, a power calculation was performed with free software (G*Power 3.1.9.2 [n]). To detect a difference of 1 grade in the histomorphology score between the treatment groups with a standard deviation of 0.5, based on a power of 0.8 and alpha of 0.05, a total sample size of 10 horses was required.

Statistical analysis and graph design were performed with commercial software (SAS 9.4m5 with the Enterprise Guide Client 7.15[o] and GraphpadPrism7.0e[p]). A p-value of <0.05 was considered significant. Testing for normal distribution was done by visual assessment of the qq-plots of the model residuals and the Shapiro-Wilks-test. Variance homogeneity in the groups was assessed by visual assessment of box and whisker plots and Levene's test (for ANOVA). The normal distributed cardiovascular parameters HR, MAP, CI and OER as well as the end tidal isoflurane concentration were expressed as mean (± standard deviation). The data that were neither normal nor lognormal distributed (histomorphology scores and the cell counts for TUNEL, cleaved caspase-3 and calprotectin) were expressed as median (min-max). For the latter, distribution free nonparametric models were used for independent (treatment and control groups) and correlated effects (time points). To correct for the variation in the number of apoptotic cells in the pre-ischaemia samples, the positive cell counts of the TUNEL and caspase stained slides were rescaled and expressed as a percentage of the cell count in the pre-ischaemia sample (relative cell count). A Kruskal-Wallis test in combination with a Dunn's multiple comparisons test was used to compare the results between the different groups at each time point, assessing the histomorphology score, the relative cell counts in percentages in the caspase and TUNEL stained slides, and the absolute cell counts of the calprotectin stained slides. For comparing the correlated different time points, a permutation test (as exact Friedman test) was used [19], with the post hoc Sidak-test for multiple pairwise comparisons, complying the experimentwise error rate. These calculations were done with the SAS macro RIBDPERM.MAC[q]. For the cardiovascular parameters of HR, MAP, CI and OER, a two-way analysis of variance (ANOVA) was performed for one independent effect (group), and the time points as repeated effect. This was implemented to compare the values between the different time points and groups, with the horses as subject effect and compound symmetry as covariance structure, taking the interaction term into account. Multiple pairwise comparisons were performed with a post-hoc Tukey test. End-tidal isoflurane concentrations, dobutamine rates and intravenous fluid rates were averaged over all time points for each horse, and a one-way ANOVA was used to compare the three groups for these variables.

Results

Anaesthetic parameters

The mean end tidal concentrations of isoflurane (ET iso) to maintain an adequate depth of anaesthesia were 1.45 (± 0.07) vol %, 1.21 (± 0.1) vol%, and 1.18 (± 0.13) vol% for group C, L and X, respectively. This was significantly higher in group C compared to group L (p=0.008, mean difference 0.24, confidence interval (CI) 0.06 to 0.41) and group X (p = 0.004, mean difference 0.27, CI 0.09 – 0.20). The mean dobutamine rate during the anaesthetic period was 0.5 (± 0.00), 0.4 (± 0.36) and 0.17 (± 0.13) µg/kg/min for group C, L and X, respectively, without a significant difference between the groups (p=0.09). The mean fluid rate was 5.0 (± 0.00), 9.82 (SD 3.14), 8.05 (SD 2.15) ml/kg/h for group C, L and X respectively. The fluid rate was significantly higher in group L compared to group C with a mean difference of 4.8 ml (CI -8.53 – -1.11, p = 0.012). Selected cardiovascular and oxygenation variables and comparison between the different groups are listed in supplementary item 2.

Histopathological evaluation

Compared to the pre-ischaemia sample, , the villous score was significantly increased in all groups after ischaemia and reperfusion (p=0.02 for groups C and L, p=0.01 in group X), but no difference could be detected between ischaemia and reperfusion (Fig 1). One horse from group X showed a very low score for the villous morphology at both ischaemia and reperfusion, with an average score of 1.2 +- 0.4 SD and 1.1 +- 0.3 SD, respectively. The haemorrhage score was 0 or 1 for all horses in the pre-ischaemia samples, and there was a significant increase of 2 to 3 grades in the ischaemia and reperfusion samples compared to the pre-ischaemia sample in group L (p=0.02 and p=0.02) and group X (p=0.03 and p=0.02)(Fig 1). There was no statistically significant difference for either score between any of the experimental groups.

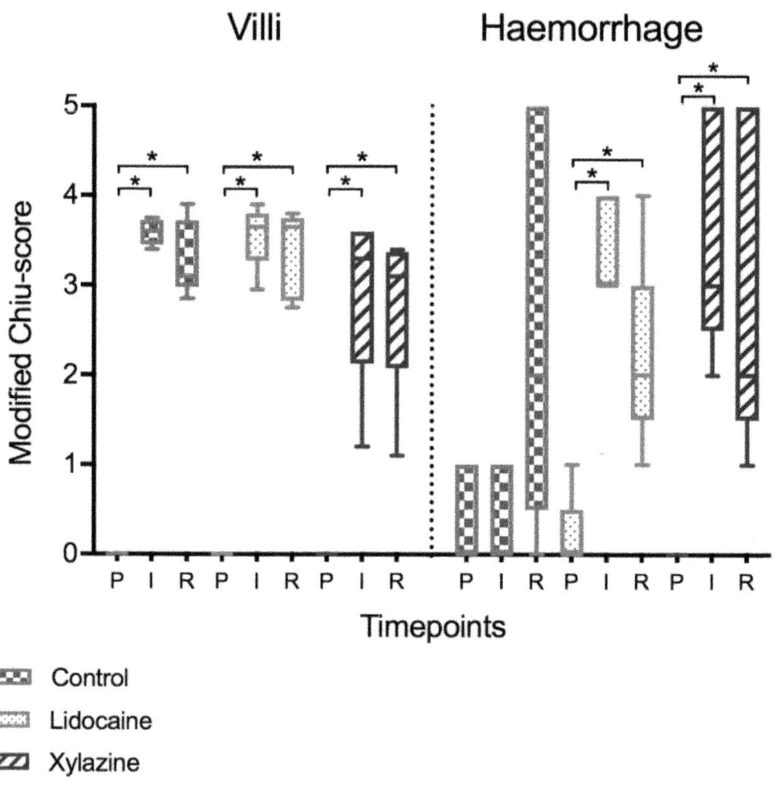

Figure 1: Box-plot diagram of the separated Chiu score for villous histomorphology and haemorrhage. The diagram displays the median, the interquartile range is represented by the box, and the minimum and maximum by the whiskers. There were no significant differences between the groups. Significant differences (p<0.05) between different time points within the groups are marked with an asterisk. P = Pre-ischaemia, I = Ischaemia, R = Reperfusion.

Calprotectin positive cells were seen in the mucosa of all slides. Compared to pre-ischaemia, all groups had a higher mucosal cell count after ischaemia (p=0.02, p=0.02 and p=0.03 for groups C, L and X, respectively) and reperfusion (p=0.02, p=0.02 and p=0.03 for groups C, L and X, respectively)(Fig 2). In group X, the cell count was significantly lower during reperfusion compared to the control group with a median difference of 6.8 cells/mm^2 (p = 0.02). In the submucosal venules, a range of 0 to 4 calprotectin positive cells per slide was found in the pre-ischaemia sample. In group L and X, the cell count had increased significantly after ischaemia and reperfusion compared to pre-ischaemia (p=0.02 and 0.03 for group L, p=0.02 and 0.02 for group X). There were no statistically significant differences at any time point between the groups. In the serosa, no calprotectin-positive cells were found in the pre-ischaemia samples. After ischaemia, only one horse in group L and one horse in group X had positive cells (2 and 8 cells, respectively). In the reperfusion sample, the cell count was 94 (86 – 117), 10 (1 – 105) and 12 (4 – 44) for group C, L and X, respectively (Fig 3). This was a statistically significant increase compared to both the pre-ischaemia (p= 0.02, p=0.02 and p=0.03 for groups C, L and X, respectively) and ischaemia (p=0.03, p=0.03, and p=0.02 for groups C, L and X, respectively). Group X had a significantly lower serosal cell count after reperfusion compared to group C (p=0.0486). No significant difference could be detected between group L and the two other groups (p>0.99 and p=0.07 for comparison with group X and C, respectively).

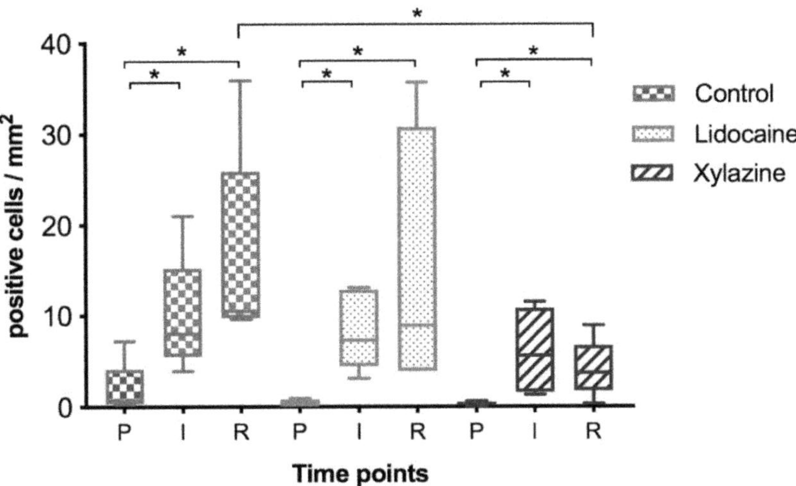

Figure 2: Box-plot diagram of the Calprotectin positive cells in the mucosa, expressed as cells per mm^2. The horizontal bar displays the median, the interquartile range is represented by the box, and the minimum and maximum by the whiskers. Significant differences (p<0.05) are marked with an asterisk. P = Pre-ischaemia, I = Ischaemia, R = Reperfusion.

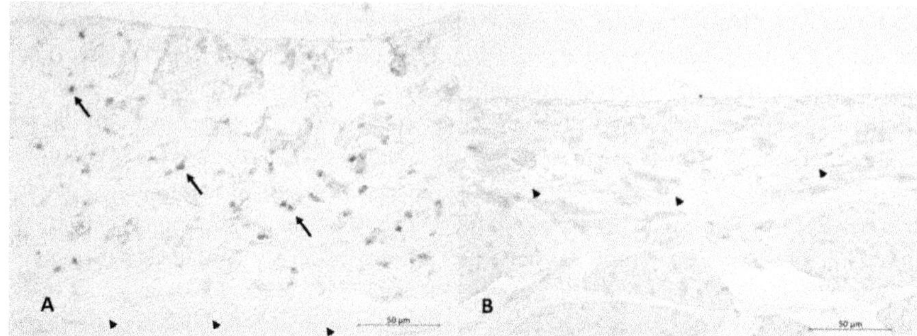

Figure 3: Microscopic images of the serosa with an original magnification of 400 (see scale bar on images). These sections were immunohistochemically stained for cytosolic calprotectin, and represent the reperfusion sample of a horse belonging to group C (A) and a horse in group X (B),The arrows indicate representative examples of calprotectin positive cells, and the arrowheads indicated the border between the tunica serosa and tunica muscularis.

The pre-ischaemic samples all revealed caspase-3 and TUNEL positive cells (Table 2). After ischaemia, the caspase cell count increased significantly in groups C and L (p=0.02 and p=0.007, respectively) (Fig 4). Group X had a significantly lower relative cell count compared to the control group at this time point, with a median difference of 227% (p=0.01) (Fig. 4). During reperfusion, the caspase positive cell counts increased significantly in all groups (p=0.02) (Fig 5). For the TUNEL positive cells, a significant increase between pre-ischaemia and ischaemia was noted in all groups (p=0.03, p=0.02 and p=0.03 for groups C, L and X, respectively), as was a significant decrease between ischaemia and reperfusion (p=0.02, p=0.03 and p=0.02 for groups C, L and X, respectively) (Fig 6). There were no significant differences between the groups at any time point. The cell debris at the mucosal surface of the ischaemia samples contained only a very low number of TUNEL positive cells (<5 cells/HPF), whereas the debris of the reperfusion samples contained many positive cells (>50 cells/HPF).

TABLE 2: Cleaved caspase-3 and TUNEL positive cells

	Cleaved caspase-3			***TUNEL***		
	Group C	*Group L*	*Group X*	*Group C*	*Group L*	*Group X*
Pre-ischaemia	10.4 (1.8 – 12.0)	4.7 (1.7 – 8.4)	5.8 (3.0 – 10.4)	15.8 (13.1 – 20.0)	11.2 (5.0 – 16.6)	8.0 (2.1 – 27.7)
Ischaemia	32.9 (13.4 – 41.4)	8.7 (5.1 – 15.2)	4.6 (3.5 – 14.2)	37.5 (22.7 – 44.0)	21.2 (9.7 – 22.3)	11.3 (10.0 – 28.8)
Reperfusion	80.9 (37.0 – 156.5)	113.3 (27.7 – 143.0)	37.8 (7.4 – 117.6)	18.7 (15.7 – 22.4)	9.0 (0.9 – 13.8)	5.9 (5.5 – 11.9)

The positive cell count for the cleaved-caspase-3 and TUNEL immohistochemistry of the different groups and time points, expressed as positive cells per mm^2 (median, minimum-maximum). Group C is the control group, and group L and group X are preconditioned with lidocaine and xylazine, respectively. *The summary per immunohistochemical stain per time point was expressed as* mean; median (± sd; minimum – maximum).

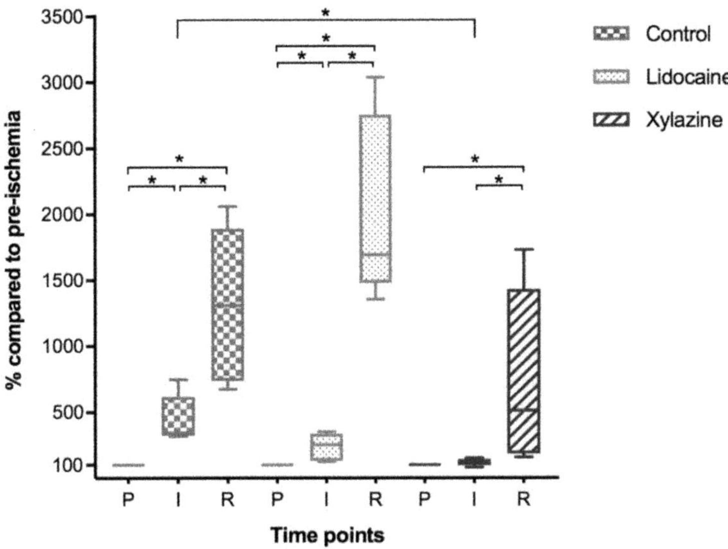

Figure 4: Box-plot diagram of the cleaved caspase-3 positive cells in the mucosa, expressed as percentage of the cell count in the pre-ischaemia sample. The horizontal bar displays the median, the interquartile range is represented by the box, and the minimum and maximum by the whiskers. Significant differences (p<0.05) are marked with an asterisk. P = Pre-ischaemia, I = Ischaemia, R = Reperfusion.

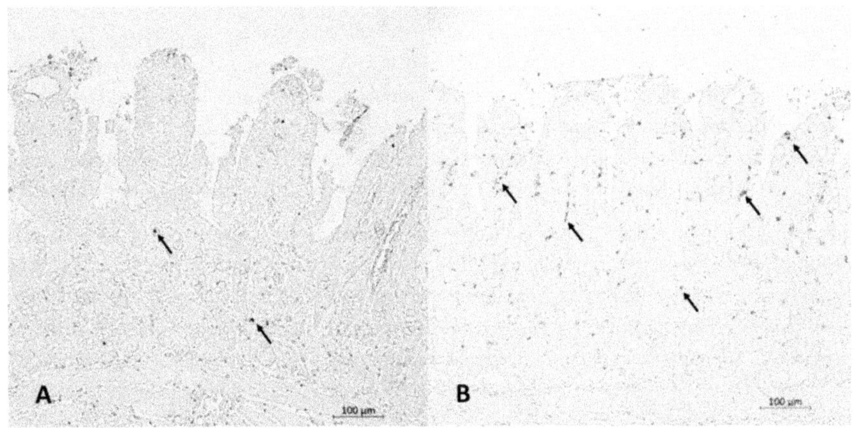

Figure 5: Microscopic images of the intestinal mucosa after immunohistochemical staining for cleaved caspase-3 in an ischaemia (A) and reperfusion (B) sample of the same horse. Original magnification 100x (see bars on images). The arrows indicate representative examples of caspase positive cells.

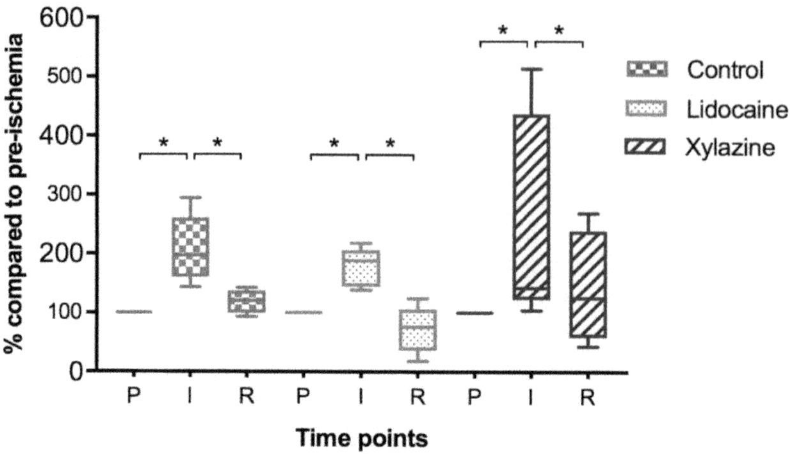

Figure 6: Box-plot diagram of the TUNEL positive cells in the mucosa, expressed as percentage of the cell count in the pre-ischaemia sample. The horizontal bar displays the median, the interquartile range is represented by the box, and the minimum and maximum by the whiskers. Significant differences (p<0.05) are marked with an asterisk. P = Pre-ischaemia, I = Ischaemia, R = Reperfusion.

Discussion

To the best of our knowledge, this is the first study investigating the preconditioning effect of lidocaine and xylazine in experimental small intestinal ischaemia in horses. No significant differences in histomorphologic changes could be detected between the groups C, L and X at any time point. The mucosal damage induced during ischaemia did not progress after reperfusion, but the number of mucosal apoptotic cells and serosal inflammatory (calprotectin positive) cells did increase during reperfusion. The main finding was that, compared to the control group, xylazine treatment resulted in a lower apoptotic cell count after ischaemia, and fewer inflammatory cells in the mucosa and serosa after reperfusion.

These results might indicate a protective effect of xylazine on I/R injury, even thought this was not supported by fewer histomorphological injury. A protective effect has also been described for the more selective alpha-2 agonist dexmedetomidine [6]. The use of xylazine for clinical cases may be more feasible, as this drug is licensed for horses and already part of many established anaesthetic regimens. Other alpha-2-agonists like detomidine and romifidine might be capable of inducing comparable effects; however, no studies on the PPC effect of these drugs have been performed so far.

The current study could not demonstrate an influence of lidocaine preconditioning on any of the tested intestinal variables. Other studies have reported beneficial effects of lidocaine on the intestine after I/R, looking at different measurements like intestinal permeability and oedema [8; 10]. The effect of lidocaine on intestinal neutrophilic inflammation in horses has not been consistent in previous studies. One author reported reduced mucosal neutrophil counts when treatment with flunixin-meglumine was combined with lidocaine administration [9], while another found no consistent decrease in neutrophil tissue infiltration [11]. The exact mode of action of lidocaine on inflammatory cells has not been clarified; however, a recent study using murine neutrophils discovered that lidocaine influences the pivotal function of neutrophil sodium channels, thereby inhibiting their adhesion and migration [20]. On the contrary, an in vitro experiment on equine neutrophils found that lidocaine did not inhibit neutrophil migration or adhesion at therapeutic concentrations, and even increased migration and adhesion at higher concentrations [21].

The MAC387 stain used in the current study to identify inflammatory cells is not specific for neutrophils, as macrophages and monocytes also express cytosolic calprotectin during inflammation [22]. However, a significant correlation between neutrophils identified histomorphologically and calprotectin-positive cells has been found in the equine colon [23]. Therefore, it is believed that this immunohistochemical stain provides a good estimate of the neutrophil count in the equine intestine. In the current study, a significant increase in calprotectin-positive cells was noted during reperfusion. Neutrophilic inflammation, initiated by the presence of superoxide radicals during reperfusion, has been indicated as a cause of reperfusion injury [1]. On the contrary, the influx of neutrophils may be part of normal tissue repair, and one cannot assume a direct relationship between higher inflammatory cell count and increased I/R injury.

The occurrence of reperfusion injury in small intestinal strangulation in horses is under debate, and it has been suggested that this does not contribute significantly to injury in clinical cases [24]. The results of the caspase-3 immunohistochemistry could indicate an effect of reperfusion in the current model, although this did not appear to cause mucosal changes on histological examination. It has been suggested that reperfusion injury may be more likely to occur in models of low-flow ischaemia, where the blood flow is typically reduced to 20% [25]. In the current study, the flow was reduced to 10%, verified by Doppler flowmetry. This model was chosen to induce significant I/R Injury without causing severe intestinal necrosis, because the latter would preclude any benefit from protective effects. The venous and arterial blood flow in clinical strangulating obstructions may depend on the type and the duration of the strangulation, and larger clinical studies on blood flow are lacking. Therefore, it remains difficult to establish a solid comparison between experimental ischaemia and equine strangulating colic.

Anaesthetic maintenance with isoflurane could have influenced the results by masking or diminishing PPC effects of the tested drugs. The protective actions of volatile anaesthetics like isoflurane and sevoflurane on I/R injury have been reported in the literature in different organs including the intestine [26]. In the current study, isoflurane could have ameliorated I/R injury across the groups, which might explain the lack of progression of histomorphological damage from ischaemia to reperfusion. Considering all horses were anaesthesized with isoflurane, this effect would be present across all groups. There is evidence indicating that the protective effect of isoflurane is dose-dependent [27]. In the current study, the mean isoflurane concentration was higher in the control group; however, this group did not have better results for any of the tested variables.

The anaesthetic protocols of this study are not feasible in a clinical situation, as general anaesthesia was induced without a sedative premedication in the control and in the lidocaine group. This set-up was chosen to avoid the influence of an additional sedative on the studied variables. Proper handling and quiet surroundings provided an acceptable quality of induction in all horses. Moreover, possible stress factors like instrumentation with the cardiac catheters were postponed until after induction of anaesthesia. The cardiac output and central venous blood gas values were not determined in the control group, therefore, CI and OER could not be calculated for these horses. When assessing the cardiovascular variables, the xylazine group had a significantly lower CI compared to the lidocaine group during ischaemia and reperfusion. However, there were no significant differences in OER at these time-points, indicating that the oxygen supply was not significantly affected by this difference in CI. Group L received more intravenous fluids than group C, which is most likely a consequence of the fixed fluid rate in group C. Because there were no histomorphological or immunohistochemical differences between these two groups, the relevance of this finding remains unclear. Dobutamine was administered at relatively low dosages of ≤0.5 μg/kg/min in all groups. According to a study assessing different dobutamine rates in horses, infusion of 0.5 μg/kg/min did not significantly affect the intestinal microperfusion [28]. Therefore, it is unlikely that minor differences in the dose range between the groups have affected the results.

One horse in group X did not show the same histomorphological changes as the others, with almost no changes in the villous structure during ischaemia and reperfusion. The micro-lightguide spectrophotometry and Doppler fluxmetry measurements indicated correct placement of the ligature, and the apoptotic cells and calprotectin positive cell counts of this horse were comparable to the other individuals of the group. Taking these observations into account, this horse was not excluded from the study.

Caspase and TUNEL positive cells could be detected in all slides, which is to be expected as apoptosis occurs as a part of the intestine's normal function. Cleaved caspase-3 is activated during early apoptosis and plays an important role in the cascade leading to DNA-cleaving, whereas TUNEL is a less specific indicator that detects the cleaved DNA that is associated with nuclear change during apoptosis or cell necrosis [29]. Considering the short time span and the lack of a comparable rise in caspase positive cells, the high TUNEL positive cell count in the ischaemia sample may represent necrotic cells rather than apoptotic cells. The decrease in this cell count during reperfusion may be explained by the observed increase in TUNEL positive cell debris, possibly indicating the separation of these cells. The low TUNEL cell count in the reperfusion sample compared to the increased caspase cell count, may reflect the difference in the apoptotic stage that is detected, because these cells may not have reached the phase of DNA cleavage yet.

Other limitations of this study are the small sample size and the use of a historical control group. Both were the consequence of limiting the amount of horses needed, and a power analysis performed prior to the study indicated sufficient power with this number of horses. We believe that the results of the historical group are comparable with the results of the test groups, as all aspects of the experiment were performed according to the same protocol and under guidance of those involved in the previous study. Regarding the comparability of the horses in the different groups, the horses in the control group appear to be younger than those in group L and X. Even though a statistically significant difference could not be detected, an effect of age on the test results cannot be excluded. Another limitation of the study design, was that only the short-term effects of PPC could be examined, and thereby limiting PPC to the early phase of protection. Furthermore, only one observer graded the histology, and the site of tissue sampling was not randomized.

The occurrence of equine strangulating colic is unpredictable, thereby precluding the application of preconditioning before the ischaemic insult has commenced. Nevertheless, there may still be blood flow to the tissue In the early stages of ischaemia, presenting the opportunity to precondition the tissue incorporated within the lesion. For the type of strangulating obstructions where increasingly more intestine is incorporated over time, the surrounding intestinal segments may be preconditioned before their blood supply is affected. Furthermore, several studies have found that pre-stenotic and remote intestinal segments also sustain injury [11; 30]. Therefore, there are several situations where the concept of preconditioning could be a feasible therapeutic strategy to reduce intestinal I/R Injury in colic horses.

In conclusion, the results of this study indicate a beneficial effect of xylazine on apoptosis rate and inflammation. A concurrent reduction in mucosal histomorphological injury could not be found, therefore, the clinical significance of these findings remains uncertain. Preconditioning with lidocaine did not have any effect on the tested variables. The results may support the use of xylazine in sedative analgesia and anaesthetic protocols for horses with strangulating small intestinal lesions. The administration of xylazine for this indication may be most appropriate in the timeframe between the diagnosis of suspected small intestinal strangulation and surgical correction of the lesion. Further research assessing the long-term effects on intestinal injury and survival is necessary to establish the value of preconditioning in clinical cases.

Manufacturer's details

a. Vygon GmbH, Ecouen,France
b. CP-Pharma GmbH, Burgdorf, Germany
c. Ecuphar GmbH, Greifswald, Germany
d. Vétoquinol GmbH, Ismaning, Germany
e. Bela-Pharm GmbH, Vechta, Germany
f. B. Braun Melsungen AG, Melsungen, Germany
g. Ratiopharm GmbH, Ulm, Germany
h. LEA Medizintechnik GmbH, Giessen, Germany
i. WDT eG, Garbsen, Germany
j. Cell Signaling Technology Europe B.V., Leiden, The Netherlands
k. Merck KGaA, Darmstadt, Germany
l. DakoCytomation, Glostrup, Denmark
m. Carl Zeiss GmbH, Oberkochen, Germany
n. Heinrich Heine Universität, Düsseldorf, Germany
o. SAS Institute Inc., Cary, North Carolina, USA
p. Graphpad Software Inc., San Diego, California, USA
q. Institut für Angewandte Mathematik und Statistik, Universität Hohenheim

Declarations

Authorship

All authors contributed to the manuscript. N. Verhaar contributed to the study design and execution, and performed the data analysis and interpretation. C. Pfarrer and S. Kästner contributed to the study design as well as the data analysis and interpretation. N. Neudeck, L. Twele and K. König contributed to the study design and its execution. K. Rohn contributed to the data analysis.

Source of Funding

The study was funded by the University of Veterinary Medicine Hannover. There were no external sources of funding.

Competing Interests - The authors declare no conflicting interests

Ethical Animal Research

The study was reviewed by the Ethics Committee for Animal Experiments of Lower Saxony, Germany, and approved according to §8 of the German Animal Welfare Act (LAVES 33.8-42502-04-17/2595)

Acknowledgements

The authors are grateful to Doris Voigtländer for her expert support in tissue processing and immunohistochemistry. We would like to thank all involved employees of the clinic for horses who contributed to the care of the horses or who gave their support in the execution of the study. Furthermore, we would like to thank the Institute for Pathology of the University of Veterinary Medicine Hannover for their technical support and helpful advice.

Data accessibility statement

The data that support the findings of this study are openly available under the following reference: Verhaar, Nicole (2019), "Preconditioning with lidocaine and xylazine in experimental equine jejunal ischaemia", Mendeley Data dx.doi.org/10.17632/bg7f74ns6z.1

References

[1] Blikslager, A.T. (2017) *The Equine Acute Abdomen*, John Wiley & Sons.

[2] Krenz, M., Baines, C., Kalogeris, T. and Korthuis, R. (2013) Cell survival programs and ischemia/reperfusion: hormesis, preconditioning, and cardioprotection. In: *Colloquium Series on Integrated Systems Physiology:* Morgan & Claypool Life Sciences. pp 1-122.

[3] Erling Junior, N., Montero, E.F.d.S., Sannomiya, P. and Poli-de-Figueiredo, L.F. (2013) Local and remote ischemic preconditioning protect against intestinal ischemic/reperfusion injury after supraceliac aortic clamping. *Clinics* **68**, 1548-1554.

[4] Sun, Y., Gao, Q., Wu, N., Li, S.D., Yao, J.X. and Fan, W.J. (2015) Protective effects of dexmedetomidine on intestinal ischemia-reperfusion injury. *Experimental and therapeutic medicine* **10**, 647-652.

[5] Kılıç, K., Hancı, V., Selek, Ş., Sözmen, M., Kiliç, N., Çitil, M., Yurtlu, D.A. and Yurtlu, B.S. (2012) The effects of dexmedetomidine on mesenteric arterial occlusion-associated gut ischemia and reperfusion-induced gut and kidney injury in rabbits. *Journal of surgical research* **178**, 223-232.

[6] König KS, Verhaar N, Hopster K, Pfarrer C, Neudeck S, Rohn K, Kästner SBR. Ischaemic preconditioning and pharmacological preconditioning with dexmedetomidine in an equine model of small intestinal ischaemia-reperfusion. BioRxiv 2019; doi: https://doi.org/10.1101/815225.

[7] Lefebvre, D., Pirie, R., Handel, I., Tremaine, W. and Hudson, N. (2016) Clinical features and management of equine post operative ileus: Survey of diplomates of the European Colleges of Equine Internal Medicine (ECEIM) and Veterinary Surgeons (ECVS). *Equine veterinary journal* **48**, 182-187.

[8] Guschlbauer, M., Slapa, J., Huber, K. and Feige, K. (2010) Lidocaine reduces tissue oedema formation in equine gut wall challenged by ischaemia and reperfusion. *Pferdeheilkunde* **26**, 531-534.

[9] Cook, V.L., Jones Shults, J., McDowell, M.R., Campbell, N.B., Davis, J.L., Marshall, J.F. and Blikslager, A.T. (2009) Anti-inflammatory effects of intravenously administered lidocaine hydrochloride on ischemia-injured jejunum in horses. *American journal of veterinary research* **70**, 1259-1268.

[10] Cook, V., Shults, J.J., McDowell, M., Campbell, N., Davis, J. and Blikslager, A. (2008) Attenuation of ischaemic injury in the equine jejunum by administration of systemic lidocaine. *Equine veterinary journal* **40**, 353-357.

[11] Bauck A. G.; Grosche A.: Morton , A.J.G., A. S.; Vickroy, T. W.; Freeman, D. E. (2017) Effect of lidocaine on in ammation in equine jejunum subjected to manipulation only and remote to intestinal segments subjected to ischemia. *American journal of veterinary research* **78**, 977 - 989.

[12] Feary, D.J., Mama, K.R., Wagner, A.E. and Thomasy, S. (2005) Influence of general anesthesia on pharmacokinetics of intravenous lidocaine infusion in horses. *American journal of veterinary research* **66**, 574-580.

[13] Pöppel, N., Hopster, K., Geburek, F. and Kästner, S. (2015) Influence of ketamine or xylazine supplementation on isoflurane anaesthetized horses-a controlled clinical trial. *Veterinary anaesthesia and analgesia* **42**, 30-38.

[14] Wittenberg-Voges, L., Kastner, S.B., Raekallio, M., Vainio, O.M., Rohn, K. and Hopster, K. (2018) Effect of dexmedetomidine and xylazine followed by MK-467 on gastrointestinal microperfusion in anaesthetized horses. *Veterinary anaesthesia and analgesia* **45**, 165-174.

[15] Reichert, C., Kästner, S.B., Hopster, K., Rohn, K. and Rötting, A.K. (2014) Use of micro-lightguide spectrophotometry for evaluation of microcirculation in the small and large intestines of horses without gastrointestinal disease. *American journal of veterinary research* **75**, 990-996.

[16] Wagner, A., Junginger, J., Lemensieck, F. and Hewicker-Trautwein, M. (2018) Immunohistochemical characterization of gastrointestinal macrophages/phagocytes in dogs with inflammatory bowel disease (IBD) and non-IBD dogs. *Veterinary immunology and immunopathology* **197**, 49-57.

[17] White, N., Moore, J. and Trim, C. (1980) Mucosal alterations in experimentally induced small intestinal strangulation obstruction in ponies. *American journal of veterinary research* **41**, 193-198.

[18] Sengul, I., Sengul, D., Guler, O., Hasanoglu, A., Urhan, M.K., Taner, A.S. and Vinten-Johansen, J. (2013) Postconditioning attenuates acute intestinal ischemia-reperfusion injury. *Kaohsiung journal of medical science* **29**, 119-127.

[19] Barg, G.L., Kraemer, D.F. and Orlando, F. The exact Friedman test and multiple comparison procedure in macro form http://sascommunity.org/sugi/SUGI88/Sugi-13-151 Barg Kraemer.pdf. Accessed on the 3d of December 2019

[20] Poffers, M., Buhne, N., Herzog, C., Thorenz, A., Chen, R., Guler, F., Hage, A., Leffler, A. and Echtermeyer, F. (2018) Sodium channel Nav1.3 ss expressed by polymorphonuclear neutrophils during mouse heart and kidney ischemia in vivo and regulates adhesion, transmigration, and chemotaxis of human and mouse neutrophils in vitro. *Anesthesiology* **128**, 1151-1166.

[21] Cook, V.L., Neuder, L.E., Blikslager, A.T. and Jones, S.L. (2009) The effect of lidocaine on in vitro adhesion and migration of equine neutrophils. *Veterinary immunology and immunopathology* **129**, 137-142.

[22] Yui, S., Nakatani, Y. and Mikami, M. (2003) Calprotectin (S100A8/S100A9), an inflammatory protein complex from neutrophils with a broad apoptosis-inducing activity. *Biological & pharmaceutical bulletin* **26**, 753-760.

[23] Grosche, A., Morton, A.J., Polyak, M.M., Matyjaszek, S. and Freeman, D.E. (2008) Detection of calprotectin and its correlation to the accumulation of neutrophils within equine large colon during ischaemia and reperfusion. *Equine veterinary journal* **40**, 393-399.

[24] Laws, E.G. and Freeman, D.E. (1995) Significance of reperfusion injury after venous strangulation obstruction of equine jejunum. *Journal of investigative surgery* **8**, 263-270.

[25] Gonzalez, L.M., Moeser, A.J. and Blikslager, A.T. (2014) Animal models of ischemia-reperfusion-induced intestinal injury: progress and promise for translational research. *American journal of physiology - gastrointestinal and liver physiology* **308**, G63-G75.

[26] Liu, C., Shen, Z., Liu, Y., Peng, J., Miao, L., Zeng, W. and Li, Y. (2015) Sevoflurane protects against intestinal ischemia-reperfusion injury partly by phosphatidylinositol 3 kinases/Akt pathway in rats. *Surgery* **157**, 924-933.

[27] Redfors, B., Oras, J., Shao, Y., Seemann-Lodding, H., Ricksten, S.E. and Omerovic, E. (2014) Cardioprotective effects of isoflurane in a rat model of stress-induced cardiomyopathy (takotsubo). *International journal of cardiology* **176**, 815-821.

[28] Dancker, C., Hopster, K., Rohn, K. and Kästner, S.B. (2018) Effects of dobutamine, dopamine, phenylephrine and noradrenaline on systemic haemodynamics and intestinal perfusion in isoflurane anaesthetised horses. *Equine veterinary journal* **50**, 104-110.

[29] Duan, W.R., Garner, D.S., Williams, S.D., Funckes-Shippy, C.L., Spath, I.S. and Blomme, E.A. (2003) Comparison of immunohistochemistry for activated caspase-3 and cleaved cytokeratin 18 with the TUNEL method for quantification of apoptosis in histological sections of PC-3 subcutaneous xenografts. *The Journal of Pathology: A Journal of the Pathological Society of Great Britain and Ireland* **199**, 221-228.

[30] De Ceulaer, K., Delesalle, C., Van Elzen, R., Van Brantegem, L., Weyns, A. and Van Ginneken, C. (2011) Morphological data indicate a stress response at the oral border of strangulated small intestine in horses. *Research in veterinary science* **91**, 294-300.

5.1. Supplementary items

Supplementary item 1

Immunohistochemical staining for cleaved caspase-3

The staining for cleaved caspase-3 was performed using the CleavedCaspase-3Asp175 detection kit (Cell Signalling Technology Europe B.V., Germany). Equine lymph node tissue served as positive control.

1. Deparaffinise and block endogenous peroxidases
   - Incubate sections in two washes of xylene for 10 min each.
   - Incubate sections in two washes of 99% ethanol for 2 min each.
   - Incubate sections in a solution of 196 ml of 80% ethanol and 4 ml of 30% H_2O_2 for 30 min.
   - Incubate sections in 70% ethanol for 2 min.
2. Wash sections in Tris Buffered Saline with Tween (TBS-T) three times for 5 minutes each
3. Heat the sections in a microwave at 800W for 20 minutes while submersed in citrate unmasking solution (pH value of 6). Cool for 10 minutes.
4. Wash sections in TBS-T three times for 5 minutes each
5. Block each section with 63 µl 1:5 Normal Goat Serum in PBS for 20 minutes at room temperature.
6. Block each section with 63 µl cleaved caspase-3 antibody diluted 1:200 in PBS with 1% BSA. Incubate overnight at 4°C. The negative control is incubated with PBS with 1% BSA without primary antibodies.
7. Let the sections return to room temperature in 30 minutes. Wash sections in PBS three times for 5 minutes each
8. Incubate with 63 µl 1:200 Goat-anti-rabbit antibody in PBS for 30 minutes at room temperature
9. Wash sections in PBS three times for 5 minutes each
10. Incubate with 63 µl ABC reagents for 30 minutes at room temperature
11. Wash sections in PBS two times for 5 minutes each and immerse the sections in PBS solution
12. Add diaminobenzidine and incubate under visual control by light microscopy for about 1 minute.
13. Immerse the sections in PBS for 10 minutes
14. Wash in cold running tap water for 5 minutes
15. Counterstain with modified hematoxylin (Delafield Hemalaun) for 1 – 2 seconds
16. Wash in cold running tap water for 10 minutes
17. Dehydrate sections:
    - Incubate sections in 70% ethanol for 2 minutes.

- Incubate sections in 80% ethanol for 2 minutes.
- Incubate sections in 100% ethanol for 2 minutes.
- Incubate sections in isopropanol for 2 minutes.
- Incubate sections in xylene two times for 5 minutes each.

18. Mount sections with coverslips and mounting medium

Supplementary item 2

Cardiovascular and respiratory variables

Table 1: selected cardiovascular and respiratory variables of the different treatment groups

Group	*Time point*	*HR (beats per minute)*	*MAP (mmHg)*	*CI (ml/kg BW/min)*	*OER*
C	*P1*	45 ± 3.6 *	61 ± 3.9	-	-
	P2	52 ± 9.5 *	79 ± 13.4	-	-
	I	41 ± 4.8 *	83 ± 20.1	-	-
	R	42 ± 3.3 *	83 ± 19.1 *	-	-
L	*P1*	33 ± 4.4 *	54 ± 7.4	37.5 ± 7.1	0.24 ± 0.06
	P2	35 ± 4.6 *	61 ± 3.5	35.8 ± 5.1	0.28 ± 0.02 *
	I	37 ± 4.4 *	67 ± 10.2	45.5 ± 12.2 *	0.23 ± 0.07
	R	36 ± 7.7 *	66 ± 18.6	46.0 ± 8.1 *	0.23 ± 0.08
X	*P1*	28 ± 1.7 *	71 ± 9.3	32.8 ± 5.7	0.32 ± 0.13
	P2	28 ± 1.7 *	78 ± 16.1	26.3 ± 6.6	0.43 ± 0.09 *
	I	29 ± 1.1 *	72 ± 11.0	33.2 ± 4.9 *	0.33 ± 0.07
	R	29 ± 1.1 *	63 ± 5.1 *	31.0 ± 4.0 *	0.36 ± 0.07

Cardiovascular and respiratory variables (mean ±standard deviation) at 4 different time points: 30 minutes after induction of anaesthesia (P1), at the end of pre-ischaemia (P2) and ischaemia (I), and at the end of reperfusion (R) for the groups C (control), L (lidocaine) and X (xylazine). Values that differ significantly with one or both other groups for that time point, are indicated with an asterisk. An overview of the accompanying mean difference, confidence interval and p-value for the significant differences between the groups, are listed in Table 2. HR = Heart rate, MAP = Mean arterial pressure, CI = Cardiac index, OER = Oxygen extraction ratio.

Table 2: overview of statistically significant comparisons between the groups

Variable	*Time point*	*Groups compared*	*Mean difference*	*Confidence interval*	*P-value*
HR	*P1*	X vs. C	-16,6	-23,82 to -9,376	<0,0001
		L vs. C	-12,2	-19,42 to -4,976	0,0005
	P2	X vs. C	-23,2	-30,42 to -15,98	<0,0001
		L vs. C	-17	-24,22 to -9,776	<0,0001
	I	X vs. L	-8,4	-15,62 to -1,176	0,0191
		X vs. C	-12,6	-19,82 to -5,376	0,0003
	R	X vs. L	-7,4	-14,62 to -0,1755	0,0436
		X vs. C	-13,4	-20,62 to -6,176	0,0001
MAP	*R*	X vs. C	-20,4	-40,03 to -0,7750	0,04
CI	*I*	X vs. L	-12,2	-23,68 to -0,8016	0,032
	R	X vs. L	-15,1	-26,49 to -3,606	0,006
OER	*P2*	X vs. L	0,15	0,01262 to 0,2846	0,0276

The statistically significant results (p<0.05) for the comparison of HR, MAP, CI and OER between the different groups, after analysis using a two-way ANOVA in combination with a post-hoc Tukey test for multiple comparisons.

6. Manuscript II

The effect of ischaemic postconditioning on mucosal integrity and function in equine jejunal ischaemia

N. Verhaar[1], G. Breves[2], M. Hewicker-Trautwein[3], C. Pfarrer[4], K. Rohn[5], M. Burmester[2], N. Schnepel[2], S. Neudeck[1], L. Twele[1], S. Kästner[1,6]

[1] Clinic for Horses, University of Veterinary Medicine Hannover, Germany

[2] Institute for Physiology and Cell Biology, University of Veterinary Medicine Hannover, Germany

[3] Institute for Pathology, University of Veterinary Medicine Hannover, Germany

[4] Institute for Anatomy, University of Veterinary Medicine Hannover, Germany

[5] Institute for Biometry and Epidemiology, University of Veterinary Medicine Hannover, Germany

[6] Small Animal Clinic, University of Veterinary Medicine Hannover, Germany

Published in Equine Veterinary Journal (2021) 00:1-11

doi.org/10.1111/evj.13450

Author contribution

- NV contributed to the study design and execution, established the surgical technique and performed the accompanying measurements as well as the microscopic examination. She contributed to the data analysis and interpretation, and prepared the manuscript.
- SK and GB contributed to the study design as well as the data analysis and interpretation.
- MHT and CP contributed to the study design and data interpretation.
- MB, NS, SN and LT contributed to the study design and execution.
- KR contributed to the data analysis.
- All authors edited or contributed to the manuscript.

Summary

Background: Ischaemic postconditioning (IPoC) has been shown to ameliorate ischaemia reperfusion injury in different species and tissues.

Objectives: To assess the feasibility of IPoC in equine small intestinal ischaemia and to assess its effect on histomorphology, electrophysiology and paracellular permeability.

Study design: Randomized in vivo experiment

Methods: Experimental jejunal ischaemia was induced for 90 min in horses under general anaesthesia. In the control group (C; n=7), the jejunum was reperfused without further intervention. In the postconditioning group (IPoC; n=7), reocclusion was implemented following release of ischaemia by clamping the mesenteric vessels in 3 cycles of 30 sec. This was followed by 120 minutes of reperfusion in both groups. Intestinal microperfusion and oxygenation was measured during IPoC using spectrophotometry and Doppler flowmetry. Histomorphology and histomorphometry of the intestinal mucosa were assessed. Furthermore, electrophysiological variables and unidirectional fluxrates of 3H-mannitol were determined in Ussing chambers. Western Blot analysis was performed to determine the tight junction protein levels of claudin-1, claudin-2 and occludin in the intestinal mucosa. Comparisons between the groups and time points were performed using a two-way repeated measures ANOVA or non-parametric statistical tests for the ordinal and not normally distributed data (significance $p<0.05$).

Results: IPoC significantly reduced intestinal microperfusion during all clamping cycles, yet affected oxygen saturation only during the first cycle. After reperfusion, group IPoC showed significantly less mucosal villus denudation (mean difference 21.5 %, p=0.02) and decreased mucosal-to-serosal fluxrates (mean difference 15.2 nM/cm2/h, p=0.007) compared to group C. There were no significant differences between the groups for the other tested variables.

Main limitations: small sample size, long term effects were not investigated.

Conclusions: Following IPoC, the intestinal mucosa demonstrated significantly less villus denudation and paracellular permeability compared to the untreated control group, possibly indicating a protective effect of IPoC on ischaemia reperfusion injury.

Introduction

Small intestinal strangulation with concurrent ischaemia can be treated successfully by intestinal resection and anastomosis. Nonetheless, there is still need for alternative strategies to reduce complications after ischaemia reperfusion injury in intestinal segments that are still vital and not to be resected.

The concept of ischaemic postconditioning (IPoC) describes the re-occlusion of blood supply in multiple cycles directly after an ischaemic event [1]. It has been shown to ameliorate ischaemia reperfusion injury in different species and tissues [1-4]. In human medicine, this treatment strategy is mainly implemented in patients with acute myocardial infarction, where IPoC can be applied after thrombolysis by reoccluding the coronary artery for several cycles of 30 – 60 seconds each [1; 5]. In the field of neurology the concept of remote IPoC has been applied, inducing short bouts of upper or lower limb ischaemia in cases of acute cerebral infarction [4]. Meta-analyses of clinical trials in people identified beneficial effects of this treatment in some of the tested variables, reporting improvement in the myocardial salvage index, stroke scores and several biomarkers [1; 4]. Most research on intestinal IPoC has been performed in rat models, demonstrating a variety of positive effects like reduced histomorphological injury, reduced apoptosis and less tissue edema [3; 6-9]. Several mechanisms have been suggested as mode of action, such as the upregulation of hypoxia inducible factor 1α or slower washout of protective factors as for example adenosine and aldose reductase [3; 6; 10].

The re-occlusion of blood supply after the resolution of small intestinal strangulating lesions may represent a feasible therapeutic strategy in equine colic surgery. There are no reports of IPoC in intestinal ischaemia in horses. Therefore, the objectives of the study were to assess the feasibility of IPoC in equine jejunum, and to assess the effect of this treatment strategy on its ability to ameliorate reperfusion injury. We hypothesized that IPoC clamping effectively reduces intestinal microperfusion in the equine jejunum, and that IPoC would ameliorate ischaemia reperfusion injury.

Materials and methods

Animals

In this experiment, 16 horses were assigned to either a group subjected to intestinal ischaemia followed by IPoC (group IPoC), or a control group subjected to intestinal ischaemia without subsequent IPoC (group C), by simple randomisation with equal allocation ratio. Two horses were excluded from the data analysis, resulting in seven horses per group. The first horse to be excluded, was the first horse subjected to IPoC. After this, small alterations in the clamping technique were made, this horse was excluded from analysis to maintain a uniformly postconditioned test group. The second excluded horse experienced severe anaesthetic problems with cardiovascular instability, prior to the surgical procedure. After exclusions, group IPoC consisted of four Warmbloods, one Thoroughbred, one Standardbred and one Icelandic pony with a mean age and weight of 10.4 ± 8.6 years and 506 ± 96 kg. Group C consisted of five Warmbloods, one Thoroughbred and one Icelandic horse, mean age was 12.6 ± 8.7 years and the mean weight 535 ± 89 kg. All research horses were systemically healthy.

Anaesthesia

Before surgery, feed was withheld for 6 hours. The horses were premedicated with 0.7 mg/kg BW xylazine (Xylavet 20 mg/mla), and general anaesthesia was induced with 0.1 mg/kg BW diazepam (Ziapam 5mg/mlb) and 2.2 mg/kg ketamine (Narketanc). Anaesthesia was maintained with isoflurane (Isofluran CPa) in oxygen, and continuous monitoring of cardiovascular and respiratory variables was performed to ensure adequate oxygenation and perfusion during the experiment. Continuous rate infusions with lactated Ringer's solution (Ringer-Laktat EcobagClickd) and dobutamine (Dobutamin-ratiopharm 250mge) were given to effect, to maintain the mean arterial blood pressure between 60 and 80 mmHg.

Surgical procedure

After induction of anaesthesia, the horses were positioned in dorsal recumbency, and a routine pre-umbilical ventral midline laparotomy was performed. Thirty minutes after induction, ischaemia was induced in a 1 meter jejunal segment by separately occluding both the intestinal loops and the mesentery with associated vessels with umbilical tape (Fig.1).

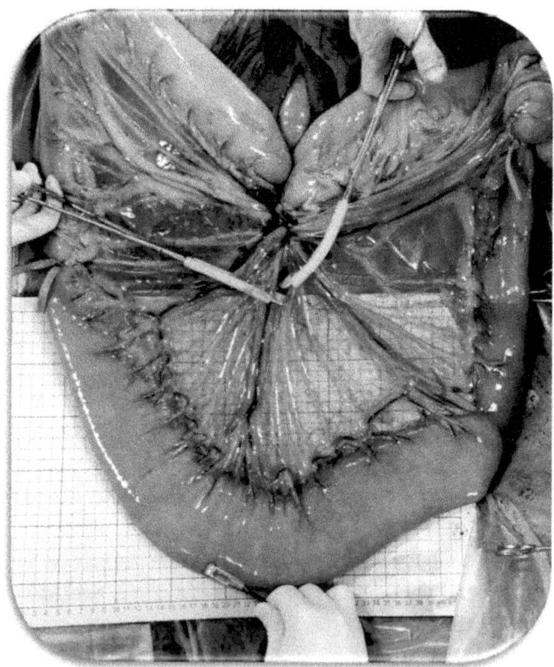

Figure 1: Photograph of the experimental set-up showing the segmental jejunal ischaemia, with clamps positioned for postconditioning. At the anti-mesenteric side of the intestine, the O_2C probe is in place to measure the oxygenation and microperfusion of the intestinal tissue.

During this procedure, the intestinal microperfusion was monitored by microlightguide spectrophotometry and Doppler flowmetry (O2Cf) [11], and the ligature was tied when the intestinal blood flow was reduced to 10 % of the baseline, creating a 90% ischaemia. After 90 minutes of ischaemia, the ligature was cut and in group C the intestines were reperfused without further intervention. In group IPoC, a delayed reperfusion was performed 30 sec after cutting the ligatures, through re-occlusion of the mesenteric vessels by clamping for 3 cycles of 30 seconds, each followed by 30 seconds of reperfusion (Fig.2). For this purpose, two large haemostatic forceps were used, the jaws covered with Foley catheters to prevent trauma to the vessels (Fig.1). During the clamping cycles, the intestinal microperfusion and oxygenation were measured continuously at 0.5 Hz. The last measurement of each clamping or reperfusion cycle was designated to determine the end effect of that cycle. After the last clamping cycle, the intestines were reperfused for 120 minutes. Subsequently, the horses were euthanized without regaining consciousness, and transferred to the institute of anatomy for educational purposes.

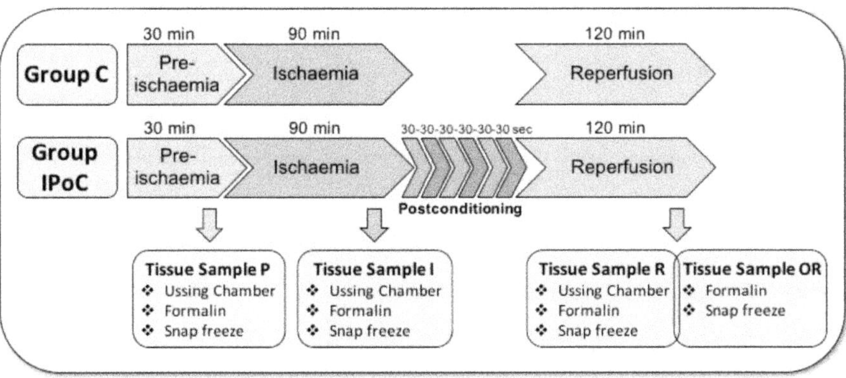

Figure 2: Flow chart of the experimental time frame with sampling time points and accompanying sample processing. Group C = control group; IPoC = group undergoing ischaemic postconditioning. The colour red represents the phases where the mesenteric vessels are occluded.

Sample collection

Full thickness intestinal segments were taken just before ischaemia (pre-ischaemia sample P), at the end of ischaemia (ischaemia sample I), and at the end of reperfusion (reperfusion sample R). A second intestinal segment was taken at this time point, just orad to the experimental segment of bowel (orad sample after reperfusion OR). In group IPoC, a mesenteric tissue sample was taken from the area where the clamping was executed. In group C, this sample was taken from the corresponding location in the mesentery.

Histology and immunohistochemistry

One section of the intestinal sample was fixed in formalin, routinely processed for histopathological examination, and stained with haematoxylin and eosin (H&E). All slides were scanned to a digital format (Axio Scan.Z1[g]), and subsequently evaluated using the accompanying software (Zen 3.0 Blue edition[g]). One section per sample was evaluated by one observer who was blinded as to the identity of the slides. Ten villi that were sectioned in proper alignment with their length-axis, were evaluated for histomorphology and histomorphometry. Each selected villus was scored for epithelial separation (EPS) and haemorrhage (HS) using a modified Chiu score (Table 1)[8; 12; 13]. The following histomorphometrical measurements were performed: villus and crypt height, epithelial-covered villus height, and maximal villus width. From these values the following variables were calculated: villus-to-crypt ratio, relative villus height compared to pre-ischaemia (villus height/pre-ischemic villus height), relative villus width compared to pre-ischaemia (villus width/pre-ischaemic villus width), and the percentage of denuded villus surface area as described previously [14]. The EPS and histomorphometrical measurements of each villus were averaged per slide. The HS was scored separately for the complete section. The mesentery samples were stained with H&E and evaluated for inflammation and injury of the mesenteric vessels.

TABLE 1: Description of the modified Chiu score assessing the histomorphology of intestinal mucosa

Modified Chiu score	*Epithelial separation score*	*Haemorrhage score*
0	Normal mucosal villi	None
1	Slight separation of epithelial cells from the lamina propria at the tip of the villus (Gruenhagen's space)	Few extravascular individual red blood cells
2	Extension of subepithelial space ± loss of epithelial cells from the tip of the villus	Mild local hemorrhage in lamina propria
3	Extension of the subepithelial space with epithelial lifting down the sides of the villi exposing a third to a half of the lamina propria	Mild diffuse hemorrhage in lamina propria ± moderate local hemorrhage (no clumping of the red blood cells)
4	Complete separation of epithelium from lamina propria to the villus base (denuded villi)	Moderate diffuse hemorrhage in lamina propria ± severe local hemorrhage, including local clumping of red blood cells
5	Loss of villus architecture and early necrosis of the crypt cells	Massive haemorrhage

Ussing chambers

The intestinal samples from 11 horses were subjected to electrophysiological and permeability measurements. The samples of the 3 remaining horses were not subjected to this analysis, due to the availability of the Ussing chambers during the experiment. One of these 11 horses showed unusually high values for tissue conductance in all samples. Therefore, this horse, belonging to group C, was excluded from further analysis, resulting in 4 horses in group C and 6 in group IPoC.

The mucosa was stripped of the seromuscular layer and mounted in Ussing chambers with a tissue exposing area of 1.13 cm^2, and bathed in a modified Krebs-Henseleit-buffer aerated with carbogen as previously reported [15]. In the absence of electrical and chemical gradients, short circuit currents (I_{SC} in µEq/cm/h) and transepithelial potential differences (PD_t) were measured through a computer-controlled voltage clamp device[h]. Tissue conductance (G_t) was determined from the changes in PD_t elicited by bipolar current pulses of 100 µA/cm^2. Fluid resistance and junction potential were measured before the mucosa was mounted, and this was corrected for during the experimental period. Measurements were performed in the pre-ischaemia, ischaemia and reperfusion samples under basal conditions, and after the addition of 10 mM alanine or 10 mM glucose to the luminal side, to evaluate the sodium-dependent alanine and glucose transport based on the response in short circuit currents. 10^{-5}M forskolin[i] was added to the serosal side at the end of the experimental period to confirm tissue viability.

In different chambers, 4 µCi of ^{3}H-mannitol[j] was added after an equilibration period of 15 min, to determine the unidirectional flux rates as a measure for paracellular permeability. Radioactivity was measured as % disintegrations/min using a liquid scintillation counter (Packard Tri-Carb liquid scintillation analyzer[i]) in 250-µL samples collected from both sides of the chamber at 15-minute intervals. Mucosal-to-serosal (J_{ms}), serosal-to-mucosal (J_{sm}) and netto flux rates ($J_{net} = J_{ms} - J_{sm}$) of mannitol were calculated from tracer appearance using standard equations.

Western blot analysis for tight junction proteins

Intestinal mucosa samples were snap frozen in liquid nitrogen and stored at -80°C until further processing. The tight junction protein levels were determined by western blot analysis in the tissue samples from horses that were included in the Ussing chamber analysis. The frozen tissue was homogenised with zirconia balls using a high-speed homogenizer (FastPrep-24™ 5G[k]) in a lysis buffer containing 250mmol/l sucrose, 20mmol/l TRIS, 5mmol/l EGTA and 5mmol/l $MgSO_4*7H_2O$ at pH 7.5 with freshly added protease inhibitor cocktail tablets (cOmplete ULTRA Tablets[l]). This step was followed by two centrifugations (2000g, 20min at 4°C and 40000g, 60min at 4°C). After discarding the supernatant, the pellet was resuspended with 10mmol/l TRIS-buffer pH 7.4 containing 150mmol/l NaCl as well as protease inhibitor cocktail tablets. Protein concentrations were measured with a commercial protein assay using Bradford reagent[m].

Two µg of intestinal crude membranes for claudin-1 and 10 µg for claudin-2 were separated by 12% SDS-Page. For occludin 2µg intestinal crude membranes were separated by 8.5% SDS-Page. Proteins were transferred to nitrocellulose membranes[n]. Membranes were blocked in tris-buffered saline containing 0.1% tween 20 (TBS/T) (claudin-1) or phosphate-buffered saline containing 0.1% tween 20 (PBS/T) (claudin-2 and occludin) with 5% fat-free milk powder.

Subsequently, the membranes were incubated overnight at 4°C with the primary antibody in TBS/T with 5% fat-free milk powder (anti-claudin-1[o]), PBS/T with 3% bovine serum albumin (anti-claudin-2[p]) or PBS/T (anti-occludin[q]). After washing, the membranes were incubated with secondary anti-rabbit antibody[i] 5% fat-free milk powder in TBS/T (claudin-1) or PBS/T (occludin), or with secondary anti-mouse horseradish peroxidase-conjugated antibody[i] in PBS/T with 2% fat-free milk powder (claudin-2). Membranes that were incubated with the secondary antibody only, served as a negative control to ensure that no non-specific signals were detected. The proteins were detected with a chemiluminescence detection and imaging system (ChemiDoc[r]), and the densitometric measurements were performed using the accompanying software. For semi-quantification of the proteins, the amount of the investigated proteins was normalized to the amount of total protein per lane. Sample analysis was performed in duplicates, and the mean of both assays was used for further data analysis. The data were expressed as percentage compared to pre-ischaemia.

Data analysis

A power analysis was performed prior to commencing the study using free available software (G*Power 3.1.9.1[s]). To detect a difference of 0.5 grade in the histomorphology score between the treatment groups with a standard deviation of 0.3, based on a power of 0.8 and alpha of 0.05 by use of a Mann-Whitney Test, a total sample size of 14 horses was required.

Statistical analysis and graph design were performed with commercial software (SAS 9.4m5 with the Enterprise Guide Client 7.15[t], and Graphpad Prism 8.3.1[u]). The data were tested for normal distribution by visual assessment of the qq-plots of the model residuals and the Shapiro-Wilks-test was performed. Variance homogeneity was investigated by visual assessment of the homoscedasticity plots and by performing Levene's test. The normally distributed variables were expressed as mean (± standard deviation), and the non-parametric as median (min-max). P-values of <0.05 were considered significant.

The ordinal variables (histomorphology score) and not normally distributed data (intestinal microperfusion and saturation) were analysed using distribution free models for independent (treatment and control group) and correlated effects (time points). A Mann-Whitney-U Test was used to compare the results between the different groups at each time point. For comparing the correlated different time points, a permutation test (as exact Friedman test) for repeated measures was used [16], with a post-hoc Sidak-test for multiple pairwise comparisons.

For analysis of the normally distributed data (histomorphometry, electrophysiology, flux rates, and western blot results), a two-way analysis of variance (ANOVA) for repeated measures was performed for one independent effect (group), and the time points as repeated effect. This was implemented to compare the values between the different time points and groups, with the horses as subject effect. The p-values were subjected to the Greenhouse-Geisser correction. Post-hoc multiple pairwise comparisons were performed between the groups for each time point with Sidak's test, and between the time-points within each group with Tukey's test.

Results

Intestinal microperfusion and oxygen saturation

Pre-ischaemia, the median intestinal microperfusion of all horses was 353 (209 – 488) Arbitrary Units (AU), and was significantly reduced to 39 (21 – 66) AU after tightening the ligature ($p < 0.0001$). At the end of ischaemia, this was 47 (32 – 60) AU. Tissue oxygen saturation was 92.5 (75.7 – 98.3) % at pre-ischaemia, and reduced to 56.7 (12.1 – 75.6) % at the beginning of ischaemia, and was 25.0 (14.2 – 44.3) % at the end of ischaemia. The intestinal microperfusion and saturation elicited by the experimental ischaemia did not differ between the groups (median difference 9 AU with $p = 0.4$, and median difference -3.1 % with $p > 0.9$, respectively).

In group IPoC, postconditioning significantly reduced the blood flow during all clamping cycles to an average of 34.5 AU ($p < 0.001$) (Fig. 3). A significant decrease in saturation only occurred during the first clamping cycle with a median difference of 47.1 % ($p = 0.02$), which was also significantly lower than the saturation during the third cycle ($p = 0.01$). During the 30 sec reperfusion cycles, microperfusion and saturation returned to the level of the pre-ischaemia measurement.

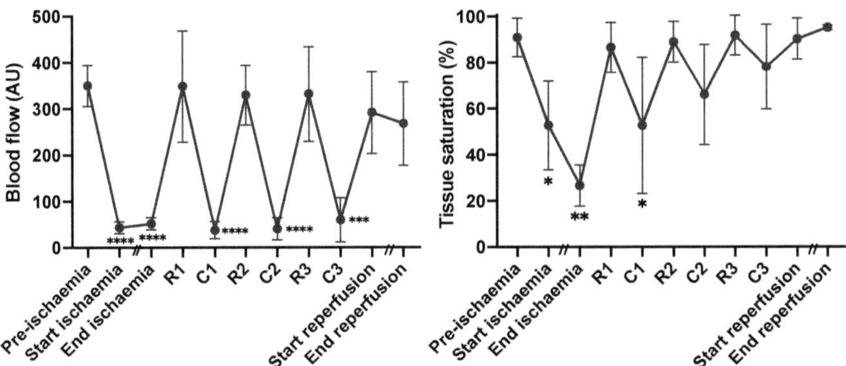

Figure 3: Diagram showing (A) intestinal microperfusion in Arbitrary Units and (B) oxygenation in % measured in the equine jejunum of horses undergoing postconditioning with three clamping (C) and release (R) cycles of 30 seconds each. Data are presented as median (min-max), time points that differ from the pre-ischaemic measurement are marked with an asterisk (= p<0.05, ** = p<0.01, *** = p<0.001, **** = p<0.0001).*

Histomorphology score

In the pre-ischaemia samples, all horses showed an EPS of 0 and a HS of 0 or 1 (Fig. 4). There was a significant increase of both scores during ischaemia (EPS $p < 0.0001$ and $p = 0.004$, HS $p = 0.001$ and 0.007 for group C and IPoC, respectively), and no change occurred during reperfusion. There were no significant differences between the groups during ischaemia ($p = 0.10$) or reperfusion ($p = 0.07$) in EPS, and the same was found for the HS ($p = 0.64$ and 0.59, respectively). Sample OR showed an EPS of 0 in all horses, and a HS of 0 in all horses except for one horse in each group with a score of 1.

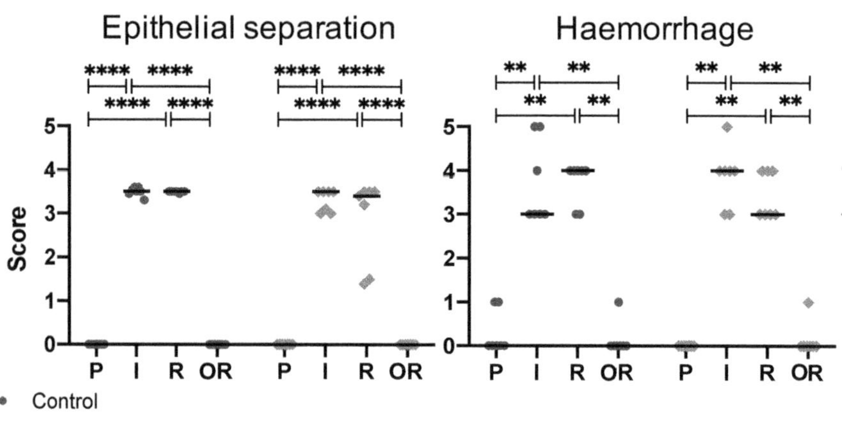

Figure 4: Individual value plot of a modified Chiu score for mucosal histomorphology during pre-ischaemia (P), ischaemia (I), reperfusion (R), and in a sample taken orad to the experimental bowel segment after reperfusion (OR) in an experimental model of equine jejunal ischaemia. C = control group; IPoC = group undergoing ischaemic postconditioning. The horizontal bar displays the median. Significant differences are marked with an asterisk (= p<0.05, ** = p<0.01, *** = p<0.001, **** = p<0.0001).*

Histomorphometrical measurements

The percentage of denuded villus surface area was 0% in all P and OR samples (Table 2). After ischaemia, this was 57 ± 15% in group C and 39 ± 5% in group IPoC (mean difference 18%, CI -1.8 to 37.9, $p = 0.09$). After reperfusion, group C and group IPoC had 49 ± 11 and 28 ± 13 % denuded villus surface area, respectively. This was significantly higher in group C compared to group IPoC (mean difference 22 %, CI 2.6 – 40.4, $p = 0.02$). The villus-crypt ratio and the relative villus height and width did not show significant differences between the treatment groups in any of the time points. These variables were all significantly affected by ischaemia, without further progression during reperfusion (Table 2).

TABLE 2: Histomorphometry results

	Pre-ischaemia		**Ischaemia**		**Reperfusion**		**Orad bowel segment**	
	C	*IPoC*	*C*	*IPoC*	*C*	*IPoC*	*C*	*IPoC*
Denuded villus surface area (%)	0	0	57 ± 15^{b}	39 ± 5^{b}	$49 \pm 11^{a,b}$	$28 \pm 13^{a,b}$	0	0
Villus-crypt ratio	2.1 ± 0.3	2.1 ± 0.3	1 ± 0.1^{b}	1.3 ± 0.3^{b}	0.9 ± 0.1^{b}	1.2 ± 0.3^{b}	2.0 ± 0.3	2.1 ± 0.3^{b}
Relative villus height (%)	100	100	37 ± 9^{b}	54 ± 16^{b}	29 ± 4^{b}	44 ± 21^{b}	89 ± 11	80 ± 10^{b}
Relative villus width (%)	100	100	171 ± 19^{b}	142 ± 24^{b}	153 ± 22^{b}	159 ± 38^{b}	113 ± 15	114 ± 7

Data are expressed as mean ± standard deviation. A significant difference between the treatment groups is marked with a matching superscript letter 'a', and significant differences of a time point compared to the pre-ischaemia measurement are marked with an superscript letter 'b' ($p<0.05$). C = control group; IPoC = group undergoing ischaemic postconditioning.

Mesentery

The mesentery of both control and IPoC horses showed hyperaemia and mild local haemorrhage around the vessels. The vessel walls were intact, and a moderate number of neutrophils was seen in and around the mesenteric vessels. No differences could be detected between the postconditioned mesentery and that of the control horses.

Electrophysiology

The values for short circuit currents and tissue conductance are summarized in supplementary item 1. Under basal conditions, the mean I_{sc} values in the different chambers ranged between -0.4 and 0.3 µEq/cm²/h. In the pre-ischaemia sample, the short circuit current increased to 3.4 ± 0.8 µEq/cm²/h in group C and 3.1 ± 1.1 µEq/cm²/h in group IPoC in response to the addition of alanine, and to 2.5 ± 0.6 µEq/cm²/h and 2.3 ± 0.8 µEq/cm²/h after the addition of glucose (Fig. 5). Compared to this time point, the ischaemia samples showed significantly less response to the addition of alanine (group C: mean difference 3.2, CI 1.26 to 4.8, $p=0.008$; group IPoC: mean difference 2.4, CI 1.2 to 3.7, $p=0.003$) and glucose (group C: mean difference 2.4 µEq/cm²/h, CI 1.2 to 3.6, $p=0.007$; group IPoC: mean difference 1.8, CI 1.0 to 2.6, $p=0.002$). After reperfusion, the short circuit current response to alanine was comparable to ischaemia, and there were no differences between the treatment groups in any of the chambers or time points.

During pre-ischaemia, the tissue conductance ranged between 13.7 – 26.1 mS/cm² in the alanine and glucose chambers under basal conditions. The addition of alanine, glucose or forskolin did not affect the tissue conductance, and there were no significant differences between the groups for any of the time points. During ischaemia, there was a significant increase in tissue conductance in both groups (group C: mean difference 5.9 mS/cm^2, CI 11.3 to 0.5, p=0.04; group IPoC: mean difference 6.0 mS/cm^2, CI 10.1 to 1.9, p=0.01) without further changes during reperfusion.

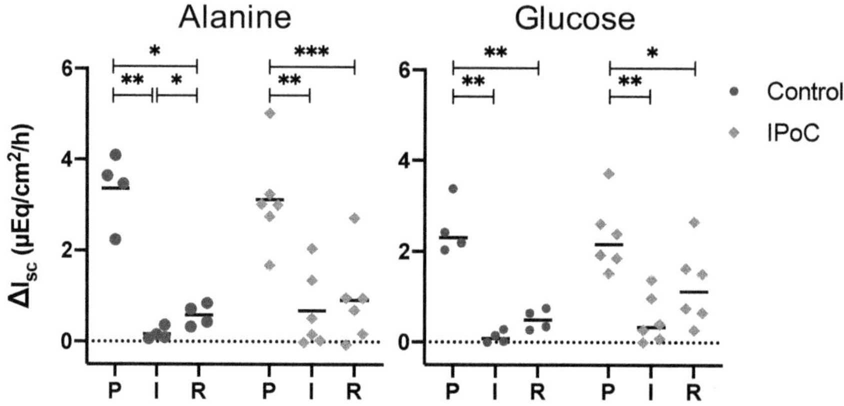

Figure 5: Individual value plot displaying the change in short circuit currents (I_{sc}) in µEq/cm^2/h measured in Ussing chambers after the addition of alanine or glucose during pre-ischaemia (P), ischaemia (I) and reperfusion (R) in an experimental model of equine jejunal ischaemia. C = control group; IPoC = group undergoing ischaemic postconditioning. The horizontal bar displays the mean. Significant differences are marked with an asterisk (= p<0.05, ** = p<0.01, *** = p<0.001, **** = p<0.0001).*

^{3}H-mannitol flux rates

Pre-ischaemia, J_{ms} was 21 ± 7.6 and 20 ± 6.3 nM/cm^2/h in group C and IPoC, respectively (Fig. 6). There was a significant increase in both groups during ischaemia (group C: mean difference -19.6 nM/cm^2/h, CI -33.4 to -5.9, p = 0.02; group IPoC: mean difference -15.0 nM/cm^2/h, CI -22.5 to -7.5, p = 0.003). Only group C showed further progression during reperfusion (mean difference -13.0 nM/cm^2/h, CI -21.0 to -4.10, p = 0.02). Moreover, group C showed a significantly higher J_{ms} compared to group IPoC at this time point (mean difference 15.2 nM/cm^2/h, CI 4.9 to 25.5, p = 0.007).

J_{sm} was 23 ± 8.5 nM/cm^2/h in group C and 24 ± 11.5 in group IPoC during pre-ischaemia (Fig. 6). Group IPoC showed a significant increase during ischaemia (mean difference -16.7 nM/cm^2/h, CI -32.5 to -0.9, p = 0.04). The reperfusion samples did not show significant differences compared to the other time points, and there were no significant differences between the groups.

Pre-ischaemia, J_{netto} was -1.4 ± 3.3 and -4.0 ± 8.3 nM/cm²/h in group C and IPoC, respectively. The net fluxrate did not change significantly over time, and there were no differences between the groups.

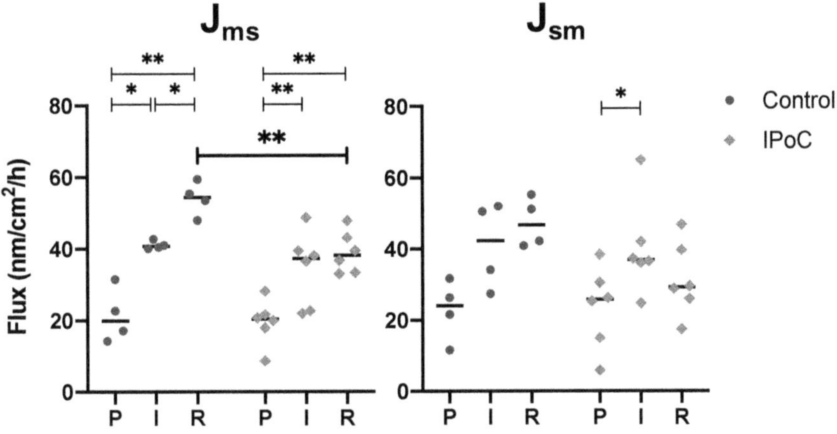

Figure 6: Individual value plot of the unidirectional fluxrates of H^3-mannitol measured in Ussing chambers during pre-ischaemia (P), ischaemia (I) and reperfusion (R) in an experimental model of equine jejunal ischaemia. Mucosal-to-serosal (J_{ms}) and serosal-to-mucosal (J_{sm}) were calculated from tracer appearance in nM/cm²/h. The horizontal bar displays the mean. Significant differences are marked with an asterisk (= p<0.05, ** = p<0.01, *** = p<0.001, **** = p<0.0001). C = control group; IPoC = group undergoing ischaemic postconditioning.*

Tight junction proteins

The claudin-1 and -2 protein levels did not change significantly during ischaemia (Fig. 7A and B). Group C showed a significantly lower protein levels during reperfusion compared to the pre-ischaemia sample for both claudin-1 (mean diff. 82%, CI 32 to 131, p = 0.01) and claudin-2 (mean diff. 68%, CI 31 – 105, p = 0.009), which could not be detected in group IPoC. The claudin-2 protein level during reperfusion was also significantly decreased compared to the orad sample in group C (mean diff. -58%, CI -98 to -18, p = 0.02). In group IPoC, the claudin-2 protein level during ischaemia was significantly decreased compared to the orad sample (mean diff. -19%, CI -34 to -3, p = 0.02).

The occludin protein level exhibited a significant decline during ischaemia in both groups (group C: mean diff. 75%, CI 43 to 107, p = 0.004; group IPoC: mean diff. 59%, CI 20 to 98, p = 0.009)(Fig. 7C). Only group C showed a significantly lower occludin level during reperfusion compared to pre-ischaemia (mean diff. 74%, CI 48 to 99, p = 0.002). Sample OR had significantly higher occludin levels compared to both ischaemia and reperfusion in group C (mean diff. -105%, CI -160 to -49, p = 0.008 and mean diff. -104%, CI -198 to -10, p = 0.04, respectively), and compared to ischaemia only in group IPoC (mean diff. -61%, CI -113 to -9, p = 0.01). There were no significant differences for any of the proteins in the direct comparison between the groups, and the orad samples did not differ from the pre-ischaemia samples.

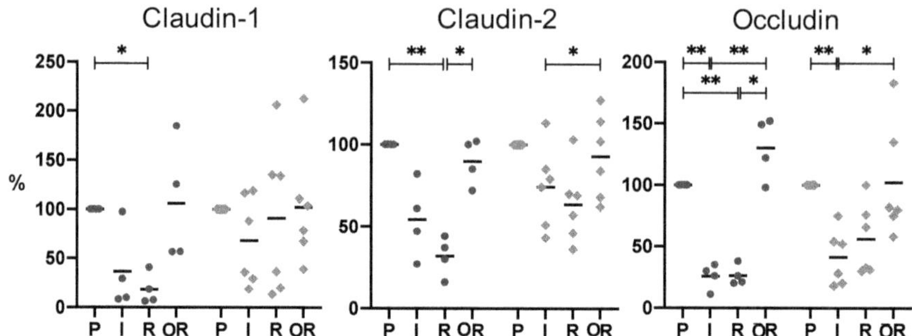

Figure 7: Individual value plot of the protein levels of (A) Claudin-1, (B) Claudin-2, and (C) Occludin analysed by western blotting of the intestinal mucosa sampled during pre-ischaemia (P), ischaemia (I), reperfusion (R), and in a sample taken orad to the experimental bowel segment after reperfusion (OR) in an experimental model of equine jejunal ischaemia. C = control group; IPoC = group undergoing ischaemic postconditioning. The horizontal bar displays the mean. Significant differences are marked with an asterisk (= p<0.05, ** = p<0.01, *** = p<0.001, **** = p<0.0001).*

Discussion

This is the first study describing the implementation of IPoC in the horse. The main findings were that IPoC clamping effectively reduced the intestinal microperfusion during all clamping cycles and that IPoC resulted in a significantly lower paracellular permeability as well as less epithelial denudation after reperfusion compared to the untreated control group. There were no differences between the two groups for the other tested variables.

In the pre-ischaemia samples, basal I_{sc} and G_t as well as the response to alanine or glucose were comparable to previously reported values [17]. The effect of ischaemia and reperfusion was demonstrated by an increase in tissue conductance and a reduction in active transport. IPoC did not affect these variables. The finding that IPoC did not ameliorate the effect of ischaemia on the short circuit current response to alanine and glucose addition, suggests that the active transport by the enterocytes was not affected by IPoC. Other IPoC studies have not investigated intestinal electrophysiological parameters and flux rates, therefore precluding a direct comparison. Both unidirectional ^{3}H-mannitol fluxrates increased as an effect of ischaemia, reflecting increased paracellular permeability. Further deterioration during reperfusion was found only in group C. Moreover, group IPoC demonstrated a lower mucosal-to-serosal flux compared to group C, indicating an effect of IPoC on paracellular permeability. The disparity between the effect of IPoC on paracellular permeability and the absence of an effect on tissue conductance, could be attributed to the transcellular pathway not being affected by IPoC. The paracellular pathway is principally regulated by tight junctions, consisting of 4 different types of transmembrane proteins including occludin, claudins, junctional adhesion molecules, and tricellulin. In the current study, claudin-1 and -2 as well as occludin levels in the intestinal mucosa were assessed. Claudin-1 is a barrier-forming tight junction important for tight junction integrity [18; 19] and the most commonly expressed claudin-protein in the equine intestine [20]. The "leaky" junction claudin-2 forms pores that regulate the paracellular movement of Na^{+} , Ca^{2+} and water [21; 22]. Following ischaemia, studies have reported decreased claudin-1, -2, -4, and -7 and occludin expression in the small intestine [23; 24]. Furthermore, zonula-occludens-1, occludin and claudin-1, -3, and -5 expression and distribution have been reported to correlate with the recovery of intestinal barrier function [25; 26]. In the current study, the control group exhibited a significant decrease in all tested tight junction protein levels at reperfusion compared to pre-ischaemia, which could not be detected in group IPoC. Due to the relatively short time frame of reperfusion, changes in protein level may reflect protein damage rather than decreased protein expression. Consequently, this result may indicate an effect of IPoC on tight junction deterioration in the mucosa. Nevertheless, no significant differences could be detected in a direct comparison between the treatment groups, although this could be the consequence of the small sample size, possibly resulting in a type II statistical error. Hence the role of tight junction proteins in the equine mucosal response to IPoC remains uncertain.

Another explanation for the reduced tissue permeability after IPoC, could be the smaller denuded villus surface area, exposing less lamina propria to facilitate leakage. A possible explanation for this smaller denuded area could be the reduced loss of epithelial cells during reperfusion or increased epithelial restitution. The difference in denuded villus area was not reflected by a significant difference in epithelial separation score. This may be explained by the fact that most ischaemia and reperfusion samples in this experimental model are assigned to grade 3 of the modified Chiu score, and the score might be not sensitive enough to detect smaller differences. Histomorphometrical assessment may be more suitable to detect smaller differences as seen in the current study. Evaluating these measurements in more detail, the denuded surface area was higher in group C during both ischaemia and reperfusion, yet the difference after ischaemia was not statistically significant. This could indicate a difference between the groups before the treatment was instituted, which may be the result of normal biological variation or disparities in blood flow in the ischaemia model used. The reduction in denuded surface area as seen during reperfusion, can imply the occurrence of epithelial restitution, or may represent a variance in the degree of injury within the post-ischaemic segment. Additional to the increase in denuded surface area, significant shortening and blunting was seen after ischaemia in both groups. These phenomena can be seen as a result of villus contraction, aiding epithelial restitution. Even though it was not statistically significant, more shortening was seen in group C during ischaemia and reperfusion. This finding accentuates the group difference in % denuded surface area, considering this is variable calculated using the villus height. A possible explanation is that the villus shortening in group C is not only due to contraction in aid of restitution, but also due to deterioration of the villus lamina propria. In summary, the histomorphometrical measurements give detailed information on the state of the villi, yet the results need to be interpreted with caution, considering statistically non-significant differences can influence the other variables, and variation in the effect of the ischaemic model complicates the analysis.

Until now, nearly all studies investigating the effect of IPoC in the intestine, were performed in rats that were anaesthetized by intraperitoneal administration of ketamine and xylazine, and subjected to complete occlusion of the cranial mesenteric artery [3; 6-9; 27; 28]. In these studies, differences in Chiu score of 1 – 2 points were found between the control and treatment groups [3; 6-9], demonstrating greater changes than those found in the current study. This may be attributed to the difference in species, anaesthetic protocol or IPoC technique. Furthermore, the difference in ischaemia model could be of significance, considering that the occlusion of the cranial mesenteric artery alone is associated with a highly variable degree of injury [29]. This discrepancy between the rodent experimental model and the clinical patient can also be noted in the field of cardiology and neurology. Even though the clinical trials performed in human patients have identified some beneficial effects of IPoC [4; 5], the vast amount of indisputably positive results reported in the experimental rodent models have not been matched, further emphasizing the importance of clinical trials.

The main limitations of the current study are the small sample size and the lack of long term effect evaluation. Furthermore, a pharmacological pre- or postconditioning effect of isoflurane cannot be ruled out [30]. This would be equally present in both groups, but it could mitigate the potential protective effect of IPoC. The elicited ischaemia injury demonstrated mild variation between the individual horses. Therefore, it cannot be completely excluded that differences between the groups are a result of a disparity in the progression of ischaemia reperfusion injury. Nevertheless, no significant differences were found after ischaemia, and the microperfusion and oxygenation results demonstrate consistent experimental ischaemia in both groups. One horse showed very high values for tissue conductance during all time points, leading to exclusion of the electrophysiological results and fluxrates from further analysis. The histology results did not differ from the other horses; therefore, the horse was not excluded from histomorphological analysis.

The use of modified haemostatic forceps proved to be a feasible technique for IPoC in the equine jejunum, and the mesentery was not affected negatively by the clamping. Different algorithms of occlusion cycles have been investigated for intestinal IPoC, ranging from 2 – 6 cycles of 10 to 120 seconds each [8; 27; 28]. It was found that shorter and more frequent cycles have the greatest effect. For the current study, an algorithm of 3 cycles of 30 seconds was elected, because this is most commonly reported in the literature [3; 6; 7; 9; 31]. Up to date, oxygenation and microperfusion have not been documented during intestinal IPoC. This study revealed that only the first clamping cycle led to significant tissue oxygen re-desaturation in this algorithm. This is most likely explained by the short time span of flow reduction, combined with a swift recovery of oxygenation during the short bouts of reperfusion. This suggests that the clamping cycle should be prolonged for a consistent reduction in oxygenation, although this may vary between species, taking differences in physiological heart rates and cardiac index into account. On the other hand, the exact mode of action of IPoC still remains unclear, and desaturation with concurrent hypoxia may not be the key mediator for the induction of its protective mechanisms [10].

In equine patients, IPoC could be implemented during colic surgery. This would not apply to intestine that is irreversibly damaged during ischaemia, but might be indicated in cases with mild to moderate ischaemic injury, where IPoC could potentially ameliorate further injury and decrease post-operative complications. From a practical perspective, clamping with haemostatic forceps may not be feasible in longer intestinal segments. In human medicine, coronary reocclusion for the purpose of IPoC is performed by use of an intravascular ballooncatheter [32], which would also not be practical during colic surgery. An alternative would be the manual reocclusion of the mesenteric vessels after release of ischaemia, or conducting the initial release of ischaemia in a decelerated manner.

In conclusion, it is possible to perform IPoC in the equine jejunum by use of haemostatic forceps, although the duration of the clamping cycle would need to be increased to establish significant desaturation in all cycles. The mucosa of horses subjected to IPoC demonstrated a reduced paracellular permeability and denuded villus surface area after reperfusion compared to the untreated control group, possibly indicating a protective effect of IPoC on ischaemia reperfusion injury. Considering the absence of a significant effect on the other tested variables, the benefit of this therapeutic strategy remains uncertain. Additional research is necessary to determine the long-term effects and the underlying protective mechanisms of IPoC in the equine small intestine.

Manufacturer's details

a. CP-Pharma GmbH, Burgdorf, Germany
b. Ecuphar GmbH, Greifswald, Germany
c. Vétoquinol GmbH, Ismaning, Germany
d. B. Braun Melsungen AG, Melsungen, Germany
e. Ratiopharm GmbH, Ulm, Germany
f. LEA Medizintechnik GmbH, Giessen, Germany
g. Carl Zeiss GmbH, Oberkochen, Germany
h. K. Mußler, Aachen, Germany
i. Sigma Aldrich, Darmstadt, Germany
j. Perkin Elmer, Rodgau, Germany
k. MP Biomedicals Germany GmbH, Eschwege, Germany
l. Roche Diagnostics GmbH, Mannheim Germany
m. Serva Electrophoresis GmbH, Heidelberg, Germany
n. GE Healthcare Europe GmbH, Freiburg, Germany
o. Affinity Biosciences LTD. Cincinnati, OH, US
p. ThermoFisher Scientific GmbH, Dreieich, Germany
q. Merck Millipore, Darmstadt, Germany
r. Bio-Rad Laboratories GmbH, Feldkirchen
s. Heinrich Heine Universität, Düsseldorf, Germany
t. SAS Institute Inc., Cary, North Carolina, USA
u. Graphpad Software Inc., San Diego, California, USA

Declarations

Authorship

All authors contributed to the manuscript and approved the final version. N. Verhaar contributed to the study design and execution, and performed the data analysis and interpretation. S. Kästner and G. Breves contributed to the study design as well as the data analysis and interpretation. M. Hewicker-Trautwein and C. Pfarrer contributed to the study design and data interpretation. M. Burmester, N. Schnepel, S. Neudeck and L. Twele contributed to the study design and execution. K. Rohn contributed to the data analysis.

Source of Funding

This study was funded by a research grant from the European College of Veterinary Surgeons and by a research grant from Stiftung ProPferd.

Competing Interests - The authors declare no conflicting interests

Ethical Animal Research

The study was reviewed by the Ethics Committee for Animal Experiments of Lower Saxony, Germany.

Informed Consent

Horses were sourced via an institutional donation programm. At the time of donation, owners gave consent for use in research and teaching generally but explicit consent for this specific study was not requested.

Acknowledgements

The authors are grateful to Doris Voigtländer for her expert support in tissue processing and histology. We would like to thank all involved employees of the clinic for horses who contributed to the care of the horses or who gave their support in the execution of the study. We are grateful to Christina Brandenberger and Henri Schulte of the Institute of Functional and Applied Anatomy of the Hannover Medical School for enabling the scanning of the histology slides.

Data accessibility statement

The data that support the findings of this study are openly available under the following reference: Verhaar, Nicole (2020), "Ischaemic Postconditioning in Equine Jejunal Ischaemia", *Mendeley Data, V1, doi: 10.17632/mxhhxpvpvj.1*

References

[1] Lou, B., Cui, Y., Gao, H. and Chen, M. (2018) Meta-analysis of the effects of ischemic postconditioning on structural pathology in ST-segment elevation acute myocardial infarction. *Oncotarget* **9**, 8089.

[2] Zhi-Qing Zhao, J.S.C., Michael E. Halkos, Faraz Kerendi, and Ning-Ping Wang, R.A.G., and Jakob Vinten-Johansen (2003) Inhibition of myocardial injury by ischemic postconditioning during reperfusion: comparison with ischemic preconditioning. *Am J Physiol Heart Circ Physiol* **285**, 579-588.

[3] Jia, Z., Lian, W., Shi, H., Cao, C., Han, S., Wang, K., Li, M. and Zhang, X. (2017) Ischemic Postconditioning Protects Against Intestinal Ischemia/Reperfusion Injury via the HIF-1alpha/miR-21 Axis. *Sci Rep* **7**, 16190.

[4] Zhao, J. J., Xiao, H., Zhao, W. B., Zhang, X. P., Xiang, Y., Ye, Z. J., Mo, M. M., Peng, X. T., & Wei, L. (2018). Remote Ischemic Postconditioning for Ischemic Stroke: A Systematic Review and Meta-Analysis of Randomized Controlled Trials. *Chinese Med J* **131**(8), 956–965.

[5] Nepper-Christensen, L., Høfsten, D.E., Helqvist, S., Lassen, J.F., Tilsted, H.-H., Holmvang, L., Pedersen, F., Joshi, F., Sørensen, R. and Bang, L. (2020) Interaction of ischaemic postconditioning and thrombectomy in patients with ST-elevation myocardial infarction. *Heart* **106**, 24-32.

[6] Wen, S.H., Ling, Y.H., Li, Y., Li, C., Liu, J.X., Li, Y.S., Yao, X., Xia, Z.Q. and Liu, K.X. (2013) Ischemic postconditioning during reperfusion attenuates oxidative stress and intestinal mucosal apoptosis induced by intestinal ischemia/reperfusion via aldose reductase. *Surg* **153**, 555-564.

[7] Li, Y.S., Wang, Z.X., Li, C., Xu, M., Li, Y., Huang, W.Q., Xia, Z. and Liu, K.X. (2010) Proteomics of ischemia/reperfusion injury in rat intestine with and without ischemic postconditioning. *J Surg Res* **164**, e173-180.

[8] Sengul, I., Sengul, D., Guler, O., Hasanoglu, A., Urhan, M.K., Taner, A.S. and Vinten-Johansen, J. (2013) Postconditioning attenuates acute intestinal ischemia-reperfusion injury. *Kaohsiung J Med Sci* **29**, 119-127.

[9] Weiwei Chu, S.L., Shanwei Wang, Aili Yan, Lei Nie (2015) Ischemic postconditioning provides protection against ischemia-reperfusion injury in intestines of rats. *Int J Clin Exp Pathol* **8**, 6474 - 6481.

[10] Krenz, M., Baines, C., Kalogeris, T. and Korthuis, R. (2013) Cell survival programs and ischemia/reperfusion: hormesis, preconditioning, and cardioprotection. In: *Colloquium Series on Integrated Systems Physiology: From Molecule to Function to Disease*, Morgan & Claypool Life Sciences. pp 1-122.

[11] Reichert, C., Kästner, S.B., Hopster, K., Rohn, K. and Rötting, A.K. (2014) Use of micro-lightguide spectrophotometry for evaluation of microcirculation in the small and large intestines of horses without gastrointestinal disease. *Am J Vet Res* **75**, 990-996.

[12] White, N., Moore, J. and Trim, C. (1980) Mucosal alterations in experimentally induced small intestinal strangulation obstruction in ponies. *Am J Vet Res* **41**, 193-198

[13] Gonzalez, L.M., Fogle, C.A., Baker, W.T., Hughes, F.E., Law, J.M., Motsinger-Reif, A.A. and Blikslager, A.T. (2015) Operative factors associated with short-term outcome in horses with large colon volvulus: 47 cases from 2006 to 2013. *Equine Vet J* **47**, 279-284.

[14] Cook, V.L., Meyer, C.T., Campbell, N.B. and Blikslager, A.T. (2009) Effect of firocoxib or flunixin meglumine on recovery of ischemic-injured equine jejunum. *Am J Vet Res* **70**, 992-1000.

[15] Wilkens, M., Marholt, L., Eigendorf, N., Muscher-Banse, A., Feige, K., Schröder, B., Breves, G. and Cehak, A. (2017) Trans-and paracellular calcium transport along the small and large intestine in horses. *Comp Biochem Physiol Part A: Mol& Integrative Physiol* **204**, 157-163.

[16] Barg, G.L., Kraemer, D.F. and Orlando, F. The exact Friedman test and multiple comparison procedure in macro form- *http://sascommunity.org/sugi/SUGI88/Sugi-13-151 Barg Kraemer.pdf.*

[17] Cehak, A., Burmester, M., Geburek, F., Feige, K. and Breves, G. (2009) Electrophysiological characterization of electrolyte and nutrient transport across the small intestine in horses. *J Anim Physiol Anin Nutr* **93**, 287-294.

[18] Saeedi, B.J., Kao, D.J., Kitzenberg, D.A., Dobrinskikh, E., Schwisow, K.D., Masterson, J.C., Kendrick, A.A., Kelly, C.J., Bayless, A.J. and Kominsky, D.J. (2015) HIF-dependent regulation of claudin-1 is central to intestinal epithelial tight junction integrity. *Mol Biol Cell* **26**, 2252-2262.

[19] Furuse, M., Hata, M., Furuse, K., Yoshida, Y., Haratake, A., Sugitani, Y., Noda, T., Kubo, A. and Tsukita, S. (2002) Claudin-based tight junctions are crucial for the mammalian epidermal barrier a lesson from claudin-1–deficient mice. *J Cell Biol* **156**, 1099-1111.

[20] Lee, B., Kang, H.Y., Lee, D.O., Ahn, C. and Jeung, E.-B. (2016) Claudin-1,-2,-4, and-5: comparison of expression levels and distribution in equine tissues. *J Vet Sci* **17**, 445-451.

[21] Amasheh, S., Meiri, N., Gitter, A.H., Schöneberg, T., Mankertz, J., Schulzke, J.D. and Fromm, M. (2002) Claudin-2 expression induces cation-selective channels in tight junctions of epithelial cells. *J Cell Sci* **115**, 4969-4976.

[22] Weber, C.R., Liang, G.H., Wang, Y., Das, S., Shen, L., Alan, S., Nelson, D.J. and Turner, J.R. (2015) Claudin-2-dependent paracellular channels are dynamically gated. *Elife* **4**, e09906.

[23] Takizawa, Y., Kishimoto, H., Kitazato, T., Tomita, M. and Hayashi, M. (2012) Changes in protein and mRNA expression levels of claudin family after mucosal lesion by intestinal ischemia/reperfusion. *Int J Pharm* **426**, 82-89.

[24] Zhang, L., Zhang, F., He, D.-K., Fan, X.-M. and Shen, J. (2018) MicroRNA-21 is upregulated during intestinal barrier dysfunction induced by ischemia reperfusion. *The Kaohsiung J Med Sci* **34**, 556-563.

[25] Inoue, K., Oyamada, M., Mitsufuji, S., Okanoue, T. and Takamatsu, T. (2006) Different changes in the expression of multiple kinds of tight-junction proteins during ischemia-reperfusion injury of the rat ileum. *Acta Histochem Cytochem* **39**, 35-45.

[26] Little, D., Dean, R.A., Young, K.M., McKane, S.A., Martin, L.D., Jones, S.L. and Blikslager, A.T. (2003) PI3K signaling is required for prostaglandin-induced mucosal recovery in ischemia-injured porcine ileum. *Am J Physiol-Gastrointest Liver Physiol* **284**, G46-G56.

[27] Rosero, O., Onody, P., Stangl, R., Turoczi, Z., Fulop, A., Garbaisz, D., Lotz, G., Harsanyi, L. and Szijarto, A. (2014) Postconditioning of the small intestine: which is the most effective algorithm in a rat model? *J Surg Res* **187**, 427-437.

[28] Santos, C.H., Aydos, R.D., Nogueira Neto, E., Miiji, L.N., Cassino, P.C., Ahmed, II, Calheiros, N.M., Garcia, M. and Silva, A.F. (2015) Importance of duration and number of ischemic postconditioning cycles in preventing reperfusion mesenteric injuries. Experimental study in rats. *Acta Cir Bras* **30**, 709-714.

[29] Megison, S.M., Horton, J.W., Chao, H. and Walker, P.B. (1990) A new model for intestinal ischemia in the rat. *J Surg Res* **49**, 168-173.

[30] Kim, M., Park, S.W., Kim, M., D'Agati, V.D. and Lee, H.T. (2012) Isoflurane post-conditioning protects against intestinal ischemia-reperfusion injury and multiorgan dysfunction via transforming growth factor-beta1 generation. *Ann Surg* **255**, 492-503.

[31] Ferencz, A., Takacs, I., Horvath, S., Ferencz, S., Javor, S., Fekecs, T., Shanava, K., Balatonyi, B. and Weber, G. (2010) Examination of protective effect of ischemic postconditioning after small bowel autotransplantation. *Transplant Proc* **42**, 2287-2289.

[32] Lønborg, J., Kelbæk, H., Vejlstrup, N., Jørgensen, E., Helqvist, S., Saunamäki, K., Clemmensen, P., Holmvang, L., Treiman, M., Jensen, J.S. and Engstrøm, T., 2010. Cardioprotective effects of ischemic postconditioning in patients treated with primary percutaneous coronary intervention, evaluated by magnetic resonance. Circulation: Cardiovascular Interventions, 3(1), pp.34-41.

Supplementary items

Supplementary item 1

Table 1: Short circuit currents

	Control group			Postconditioning group		
	Pre-ischaemia	*Ischaemia*	*Reperfusion*	*Pre-ischaemia*	*Ischaemia*	*Reperfusion*
Basal (alanine)	-0.26 ± 0.2	0.32 ± 0.06	-0.019 ± 0.02	-0.45 ± 0.6	0.28 ± 0.1	0.017 ± 0.1
Alanine	3.4 ± 0.8	0.17 ± 0.1	0.58 ± 0.2	3.1 ± 1.1	0.68 ± 0.8	0.9 ± 1.0
Forskolin	0.56 ± 0.4	0.25 ± 0.08	0.59 ± 0.2	0.61 ± 0.4	0.32 ± 0.3	0.74 ± 0.6
Basal (glucose)	-0.15 ± 0.29	0 ± 0.07	0.033 ± 0.1	-0.39 ± 0.4	0.032 ± 0.08	0.06 ± 0.2
Glucose	2.5 ± 0.6	0.11 ± 0.1	0.5 ± 0.2	2.3 ± 0.8	0.52 ± 0.5	1.2 ± 0.9
Forskolin	0.52 ± 0.4	0.058 ± 0.08	0.38 ± 0.2	0.61 ± 0.5	0.13 ± 0.05	0.61 ± 0.4

Table 1 demonstrates the short circuit current in μEq/cm²/h measured in Ussing chambers in intestinal mucosa from horses undergoing ischaemic postconditioning and an untreated control group. The basal values represent the short circuit currents in the alanine and glucose chambers before the addition of these substances (mean ± SD). The measurement after addition of alanine, glucose, or forskolin is expressed in mean change compared to the basal measurement.

Table 2: Tissue conductance

	Control group			Postconditioning group		
	Pre-ischaemia	*Ischaemia*	*Reperfusion*	*Pre-ischaemia*	*Ischaemia*	*Reperfusion*
Basal (alanine)	16.2 ± 1.7	27.6 ± 1.6[a]	26.3 ± 4.0	17.8 ± 4.4	22.9 ± 2.6[a]	24.6 ± 1.5
Alanine	0.2 ± 0.6	-1.3 ± 0.1[b]	-0.5 ± 0.2	0.2 ± 0.4	-0.1 ± 1[b]	0.3 ± 1.4
Forskolin	0.3 ± 0.3	0.5 ± 0.2	0.1 ± 0.3	0.4 ± 0.5	0.6 ± 0.8	0.4 ± 0.7
Basal (glucose)	15.5 ± 0.8	21.4 ± 2.9	25.1 ± 4.2	17.5 ± 3.4	23.5 ± 5.0	22.6 ± 0.6
Glucose	0.2 ± 0.3	0.5 ± 1.0	-1.1 ± 1.4	0.2 ± 0.3	-0.2 ± 0.4	0.0 ± 0.6
Forskolin	0.5 ± 0.3	0.6 ± 1.6	0.2 ± 0.5	0.6 ± 0.4	0.1 ± 0.2	-0.1 ± 0.6

Table 2 demonstrates the tissue conductance in mS/cm² measured in Ussing chambers in intestinal mucosa from horses undergoing ischaemic postconditioning and an untreated control group. The basal values display the tissue conductance in the alanine and glucose chambers before the addition of these substances (mean ± SD). The values for tissue conductance after addition of alanine, glucose, or forskolin, are expressed in mean change compared to basal measurement.

7. Manuscript III

Ischaemic postconditioning reduces apoptosis in experimental jejunal ischaemia in horses

Nicole Verhaar[1], Nicole de Buhr[2,3], Maren von Köckritz-Blickwede[2,3], Marion Hewicker-Trautwein[4], Christiane Pfarrer[5], Gemma Mazzuoli-Weber[6], Henri Schulte[7], Sabine Kästner[1,8]

[1] Clinic for Horses, University of Veterinary Medicine Hannover, Germany

[2] Department of Biochemistry, University of Veterinary Medicine Hannover, Germany

[3] Research Center for Emerging Infections and Zoonoses (RIZ)

[4] Institute of Pathology, University of Veterinary Medicine Hannover, Germany

[5] Institute for Anatomy, University of Veterinary Medicine Hannover, Germany

[6] Institute for Physiology and Cell Biology, University of Veterinary Medicine Hannover, Germany

[7] Institute of Functional and Applied Anatomy, Hannover Medical School Hannover, Germany

[8] Small Animal Clinic, University of Veterinary Medicine Hannover, Germany

Published in BMC Veterinary Research (2021) 17:175

doi.org/10.1186/s12917-021-02877-y

Author contribution

- NV contributed to the study design and execution including the immunohistochemical staining, the microscopic examinations, and establishment of the enzyme assays. NV performed the data analysis, contributed to the interpretation and prepared the manuscript.
- NdB, GMW and SK contributed to the study design as well as the data analysis and interpretation.
- MKB, MHT and CP contributed to the study design and data interpretation.
- HS contributed to the study execution and data analysis.
- All authors edited or contributed to the manuscript.

Abstract

Background: Ischaemic postconditioning (IPoC) refers to brief periods of reocclusion of blood supply following an ischaemic event. This has been shown to ameliorate ischaemia reperfusion injury in different tissues, and it may represent a feasible therapeutic strategy for ischaemia reperfusion injury following strangulating small intestinal lesions in horses. The objective of this study was to assess the degree cell death, inflammation, oxidative stress, and heat shock response in an equine experimental jejunal ischaemia model with and without IPoC.

Methods: In this randomized, controlled, experimental in vivo study, 14 horses were evenly assigned to a control group and a group subjected to IPoC. Under general anaesthesia, segmental ischaemia with arterial and venous occlusion was induced in 1.5 m jejunum. Following ischaemia, the mesenteric vessels were repeatedly re-occluded in group IPoC only. Full thickness intestinal samples and blood samples were taken at the end of the pre-ischaemia period, after ischaemia, and after 120 min of reperfusion. Immunohistochemical staining or enzymatic assays were performed to determine the selected variables.

Results: The mucosal cleaved-caspase-3 and TUNEL cell counts were significantly increased after reperfusion in the control group only. The cleaved-caspase-3 cell count was significantly lower in group IPoC after reperfusion compared to the control group. After reperfusion, the tissue myeloperoxidase activity and the calprotectin positive cell counts in the mucosa were increased in both groups, and only group IPoC showed a significant increase in the serosa. Tissue malondialdehyde and superoxide dismutase as well as blood lactate levels showed significant progression during ischaemia or reperfusion. The nuclear immunoreactivity of Heat shock protein-70 increased significantly during reperfusion. None of these variables differed between the groups. The neuronal cell counts in the myenteric plexus ganglia were not affected by the ischaemia model.

Conclusions: A reduced apoptotic cell count was found in the group subjected to IPoC. None of the other tested variables were significantly affected by IPoC. Therefore, the clinical relevance and possible protective mechanism of IPoC in equine intestinal ischaemia remains unclear. Further research on the mechanism of action and its effect in clinical cases of strangulating colic is needed.

Background

Strangulating small intestinal lesions in horses can be effectively treated by small intestinal resection. Nevertheless, there is still a need for additional therapeutic strategies, as some cases are not amenable to intestinal resection, and concurrent disease such as post-operative ileus and adhesions are associated with high mortality rates (1, 2). These complications can result from intestinal damage during ischaemia or due to reperfusion injury (3, 4). During reperfusion, the formations of reactive oxygen species can induce oxidative injury and neutrophilic inflammation, leading to mucosal and seromuscular damage (2, 5-7). This may also affect the intestinal neurons, contributing to postoperative motility disorders (8, 9).

Ischaemic postconditioning (IPoC) refers to brief periods of reocclusion of blood supply following an ischaemic event, thereby preventing immediate reperfusion (10). This principle was first described in the myocardium (11), followed by its application in many tissues including the small intestine, kidney, liver and brain (10, 12). Most research assessing the effect of IPoC on intestinal ischaemia/reperfusion (I/R) injury, has been performed in laboratory animals by use of an experimental model occluding the cranial mesenteric artery. Many different variables for intestinal ischaemia reperfusion injury have been investigated in these studies, where intestinal IPoC was most commonly associated with decreased histomorphological damage (13-21). Moreover, reduced apoptosis, less oxidative stress and neutrophil activation, as well as higher superoxide dismutase or glutathion levels have been reported in groups subjected to IPoC (14-21). It has been suggested that the reocclusion delays the washout of mediators such as adenosine and bradykinin, which may elicit a protective response (10, 22). Many signalling pathways have been indicated to mediate the effect of IPoC; however, the exact mechanism of action of IPoC remains unknown (12, 22). Heat shock proteins (HSPs) are molecular chaperones for protein repair that are upregulated in response to a variety of noxious stimuli (23). Especially the HSP-70 family has been shown to play a protective role in the intestine, with upregulation after intestinal I/R in different animal models (24, 25), and reduced intestinal necrosis associated with higher HSP-70 levels (26). Furthermore, the upregulation of HSP-70 has been reported after remote conditioning and ischaemic preconditioning in the brain, spinal cord and heart (27-29). Until now, the role of HSP-70 has not been assessed in tissues undergoing IPoC or in experimental equine jejunal ischaemia.

A recent study investigating IPoC in experimental jejunal ischaemia in horses, found lower mucosal permeability and less epithelial denudation in the group undergoing IPoC (30). IPoC could represent a feasible technique for clinical cases of strangulating colic; however, more information on the effect of IPoC in the ischaemic equine intestine is needed. The objective of this study was to assess the degree of cell death, inflammation, oxidative stress, and heat shock response during experimental small intestinal ischaemia in horses subjected to IPoC and horses undergoing normal reperfusion. We hypothesized that IPoC would decrease apoptosis, inflammation, neuronal cell death, and oxidative stress in the equine intestine after I/R injury. Furthermore, we hypothesised that IPoC would be accompanied by an increased heat shock response.

Results

Cell apoptosis

To quantify the number of apoptotic cells in the mucosa, paraffin sections were immunohistochemically stained for cleaved-caspase-3. The cells exhibiting positive staining were enterocytes, stromal cells and inflammatory cells. During pre-ischaemia, the control group (group C) exhibited 10.2 ± 5.2 cleaved-caspase-3 positive cells/mm^2, and group IPoC 4.4 ± 1.6 (Fig 1A). During ischaemia, group IPoC showed a significant increase in positive cells (mean difference -9.8 cells/mm^2, CI -19 to -0.6, p = 0.04), without further progression during reperfusion. Group C showed a significant increase during reperfusion compared to pre-ischaemia (mean diff. -92.2 cells/mm^2, CI -140 to -44, p = 0.002), ischaemia (mean diff. -86.8 cells/mm^2, CI -133 to -41, p = 0.002), and the sample that was taken proximal to the ischaemic segment at the time point of reperfusion (Sample PR) (mean diff. 92.5 cells/mm^2, CI 33 to 153, p = 0.006). There were no significant differences between both groups during pre-ischaemia and ischaemia; however, the cell count was significantly lower in group IPoC after reperfusion (mean diff. 57.7 cell/mm^2, CI 1.2 to 114, p = 0.04). As additional marker for apoptosis and necrosis, a TUNEL assay was performed. During pre-ischaemia, the TUNEL positive cell count was 20.5 ± 9.3 cells/mm^2 in group C, and 27.4 ± 8.1 in group IPoC (Fig 1B). The increase in positive cells during ischaemia was not statistically significant. Group C exhibited a significant increase in the reperfusion sample compared to pre-ischaemia with a mean difference of 43.6 cells/mm^2 (CI -85.8 to -1.4, p = 0.04). On the contrary, group IPoC did not show an increase during reperfusion. In both groups, the TUNEL positive cell counts were significantly lower in the PR samples compared to both ischaemia (group C: mean diff. 24.5 cells/mm^2, CI 0.9 to 48, p = 0.04; group IPoC: mean diff. 18.8 cells/mm^2, CI 6.9 to 31, p = 0.006) and reperfusion (group C: mean diff. 51.3 cells/mm^2, CI 6.8 to 96, p = 0.03; group IPoC: mean diff. 24.1 cells/mm^2, CI 3.3 to 45, p = 0.03). There were no significant differences between the groups for any of the time points.

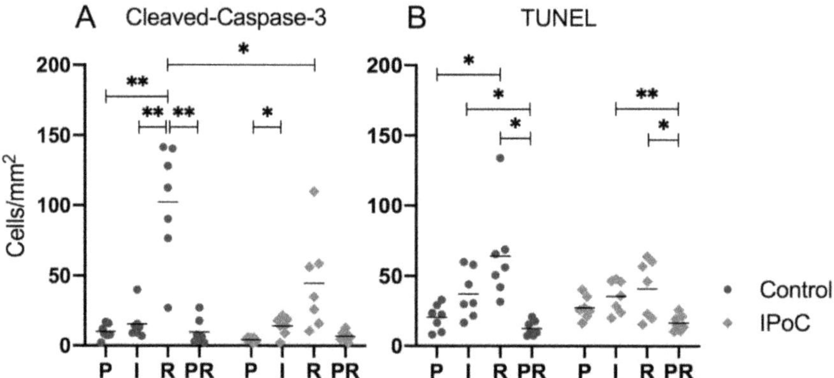

Fig 1. Cleaved-caspase- and TUNEL positive cell counts in the intestinal mucosa. Individual value plots of positive cell counts in cells/mm^2 after immunohistochemical staining for cleaved-caspase-3 (A) and TUNEL (B) in the small intestinal mucosa from horses subjected to postconditioning (IPoC) and an untreated control group. The horizontal bar displays the mean. Significant differences are marked with an asterisk (p<0.05; ** p<0.01). P = Pre-ischaemia, I = Ischaemia, R = Reperfusion, PR = proximal intestinal segment after reperfusion.*

Inflammatory cells

To assess the inflammatory cell count in the intestinal tissue, the sections were immunohistochemically stained for cytosolic calprotectin, which is present in neutrophils, monocytes and macrophages. There were no significant differences between the two groups for any of the time points or intestinal sections. In the mucosa of both groups, the reperfusion sample showed a significantly higher cell count compared to all other time points (Fig. 2 and 3). In the submucosa and muscularis propria, there were no significant changes over time, except for a higher submucosal cell count during reperfusion compared to pre-ischaemia in group C (mean diff. -4.1 cells/mm^2, CI -7.8 to -0.5, p = 0.03). In the serosa, no significant differences could be detected between the time points in group C. However, group IPoC showed significantly higher cell counts in the reperfusion and PR sample, compared to both pre-ischaemia and ischaemia (Fig. 2).

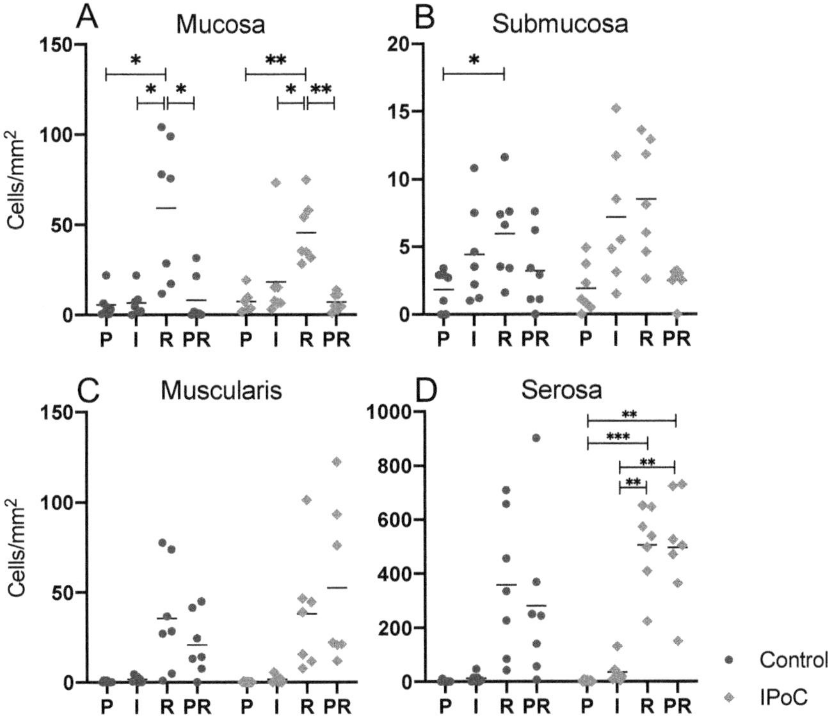

Fig 2. Calprotectin positive cell counts in the intestine. Individual value plots of the positive cell counts in cells/mm^2 after immunohistochemical staining for cytosolic calprotectin in the mucosa (A), submucosa (B), muscularis (C) and serosa (D) of an untreated control group and a group subjected to IPoC. There were no significant differences between the groups. The horizontal bar displays the mean. Significant differences between the time points are marked with an asterisk (p<0.05; ** p<0.01; *** p<0.001). P = Pre-ischaemia, I = Ischaemia, R = Reperfusion, PR = proximal intestinal segment sampled after reperfusion.*

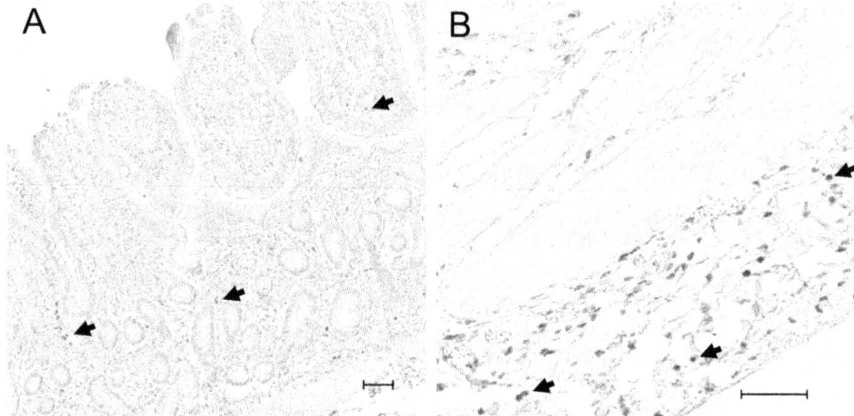

Fig 3. Calprotectin immunoreactivity in the small intestine. Microscopic images of immunohistochemical staining for cytosolic calprotectin in the mucosa (A) and serosa (B) from the same intestinal sample taken after reperfusion, illustrating the intense positive staining of inflammatory cells in these locations (arrows). The scale bar represents 50 µm.

Heat Shock Protein-70

Immunohistochemistry for inducible HSP-70 was performed as an indicator for the heat shock response. Mainly enterocytes and inflammatory cells exhibited positive staining. During pre-ischaemia, the enterocytes of the crypts and the villus base exhibited no nuclear staining, and merely weak – mild staining of the cytoplasm, whereas the villus apex showed more staining of the enterocyte cytoplasm (1, 1 – 2) and nucleus (1, 0 – 2). There was no significant increase of the total cytoplasm and nucleus score during ischaemia (Fig 4A). Yet reperfusion exhibited a significant rise in total nucleus score compared to both pre-ischaemia ($p = 0.03$ and 0.004 for group C and IPoC, respectively) and ischaemia ($p = 0.02$ for both groups) (Figs 4B and 5). The total cytoplasm score did not significantly change during reperfusion. No differences between the treatment groups could be detected. When comparing the total cytoplasm score with the nucleus score for each time point, the cytoplasm staining was significantly higher than that of the nuclei at all time points except for the reperfusion time point. The staining of the muscularis was mild to moderate during pre-ischaemia, and did not change significantly over time (Fig 4C).

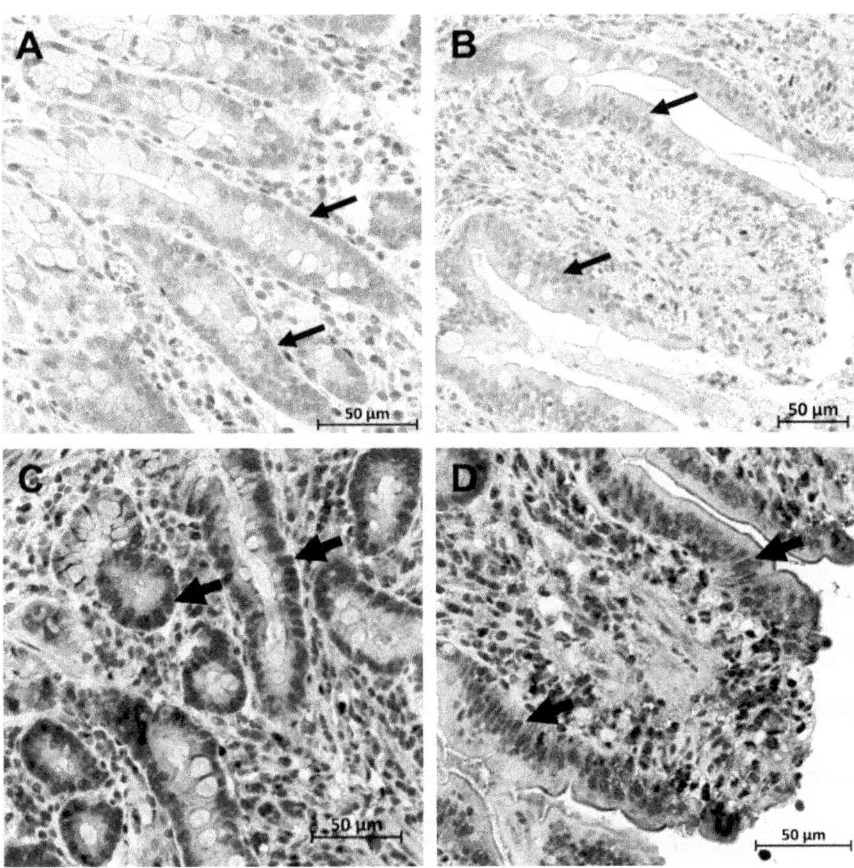

Fig 4. Heat Shock Protein-70 immunoreactivity score. Individual value plots of a semi-quantitative score assessing the immunoreactivity after immunohistochemical staining for Heat Shock Protein-70 of the small intestine from horses subjected to postconditioning (IPoC) and an untreated control group. The mucosal cytoplasm (A), the nuclei (B) and the muscularis propria (C) were scored separately. The horizontal bar displays the mean. Significant differences are marked with an asterisk (p<0.05; ** p<0.01). P = Pre-ischaemia, I = Ischaemia, R = Reperfusion, PR = proximal intestinal segment after reperfusion.*

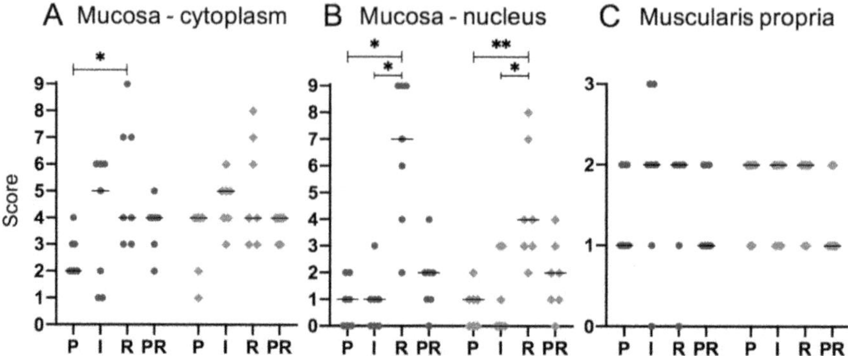

Fig 5. Heat Shock Protein-70 immunoreactivity in the small intestinal mucosa. Microscopic images of the crypts and villi of the small intestinal mucosa after immunohistochemical staining for Heat Shock Protein-70. Panels A and B are from an ischaemic sample, and C and D are from the reperfusion sample of the same horse, illustrating an increase in immunoreactivity. Representative examples of the stained enterocyte nuclei are marked (narrow arrow for weak stained nuclei, broad arrows for the intensely stained nuclei), the enterocyte cytoplasm shows a mild to moderate staining.

Myenteric plexus

To assess the neuronal cell count, Hu and NOS were immunohistochemically stained in a whole mount preparation of the myenteric plexus. Hu is an RNA binding protein commonly expressed in all enteric neurons, thus used as a pan-neuronal marker (31). NOS is highly prevalent in interneurons and inhibitory motor neurons for the synthesis of nitric oxide as inhibitory neurotransmitter (9, 32). A wide range in ganglion size was found, with a median of 37 (3 – 291) Hu-immunoreactive neurons in group C and 25 (2 – 321) in group IPoC (Fig 6A and C). The NOS stained neurons exhibited a comparable variance, with 8 (0 – 67) positive neurons per ganglion in group C and 5 (0 – 64) in group IPoC (Fig 6B and D), representing 21 and 22% of the total neuronal count, respectively. No changes could be detected after ischaemia or reperfusion, and there were no significant differences in absolute or relative cell counts between the groups (Fig 6). The Hu- and NOS-positive staining was localized in the neuronal cytoplasm, and a translocation of Hu-immunoreactivity to the nucleus could not be observed in any of the samples (Fig 7).

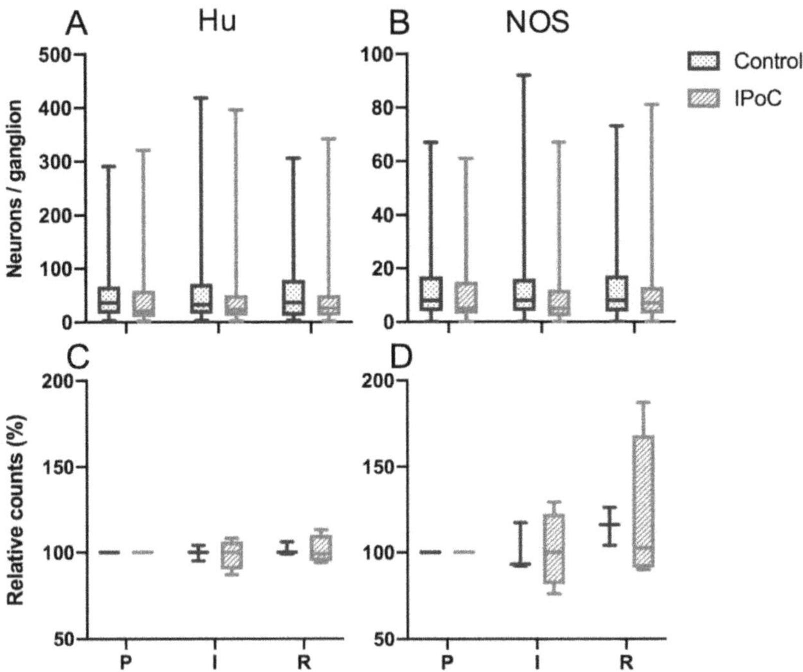

Fig 6. Hu and NOS stained neuronal counts in the myenteric plexus. Boxplot diagram of the Hu and NOS immunohistochemistry results. The left panels display the absolute and relative counts of the Hu stained neurons, and the right panels the NOS. The horizontal bar displays the median, the interquartile range is represented by the box, and the minimum and maximum by the whisker plots. IPoC = group undergoing postconditioning; P = pre-ischaemia; I = ischaemia; R = reperfusion.

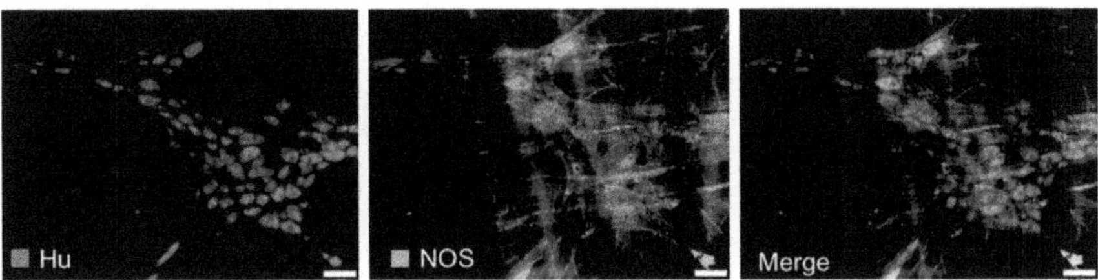

Fig 7. Hu and NOS immunoreactivity in the myenteric plexus. Fluorescence microscopy image of a ganglion in the myenteric plexus, displaying the cytoplasmic staining for Hu-positive neurons (red), and NOS-positive neurons (green). Scale bar 100 µm.

Tissue levels of superoxide dismutase, myeloperoxidase and malondialdehyde

Superoxide dismutase (SOD) and malondialdehyde (MDA) as markers for oxidative stress and myeloperoxidase (MPO) as indicator for neutrophilic inflammation were determined in full thickness intestinal tissue samples including mucosa and serosa. For these variables, no differences could be detected between the groups for any of the time points. During pre-ischaemia, the SOD activity was 1.8 (± 0.4) and 2.0 (± 0.6) units/mg protein in group C and IPoC, respectively (Fig 8A). A significant decrease was observed in both groups during ischaemia (group C: mean diff. 0.52, CI 0.11 to 1.0, p = 0.04; group IPoC: mean diff. 0.64, CI 0.13 to 1.2, p = 0.01), without further progression during reperfusion. MDA content was 3.4 (± 1.3) nM/mg protein in group C and 4.2 (± 5.7) in group IPoC during pre-ischaemia (Fig 8B). No significant increase could be detected during ischaemia and reperfusion. The PR sample did show significantly lower values compared to ischaemia in group C (mean diff. 4.6, CI 0.2 to 8.9, p = 0.04) and compared to reperfusion in group IPoC (mean diff. 4.9, CI 0.3 to 9.5, p = 0.03). Barely any MPO activity was detected during pre-ischaemia, with a median of 0 (0 – 3.5) and 0 (0 – 0.9) units/mg protein for group C and IPoC, respectively (Fig 8C). The activity was significantly higher during ischaemia in group IPoC, compared to pre-ischaemia (median diff. 2.1, p = 0.02) and the PR sample (median diff. 2.1, p = 0.004). In both groups, the PR sample showed significantly less MPO activity compared to the reperfusion segment (group C: median diff. 4.5, p = 0.04; group IPoC: median diff. 2.8, p = 0.04)

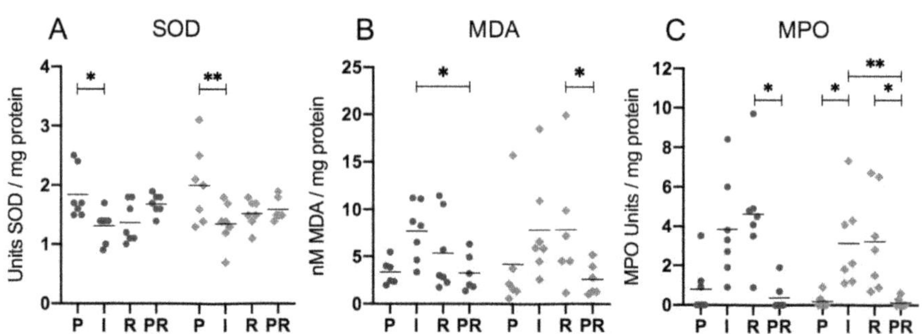

Fig 8. SOD and MPO activity and MDA content in the small intestine. Individual value plots of superoxide dismutase activity (A), malondialdehyde content (B), and myeloperoxidase activity (C) measured in full thickness intestinal tissue from horses subjected to postconditioning (IPoC) and an untreated control group. The horizontal bar displays the median. Significant differences are marked with an asterisk (p<0.05; ** p<0.01;). P = Pre-ischaemia, I = Ischaemia, R = Reperfusion, PR = proximal intestinal segment after reperfusion.*

Plasma levels of lactate, lactate-dehydrogenase and creatine-kinase

To determine the level of systemic oxidative stress, lactate, lactate dehydrogenase (LDH) and creatine kinase (CK) were measured in arterial (lactate) and venous (LDH and CK) blood samples. Pre-ischaemia, the lactate level was 1.1 (0.8 – 1.4), LDH 151 (123 – 206) and CK was 122 (88 – 180) mmol/l in group C. Plasma levels in group IPoC were 1.6 (0.9 – 2.2), 147 (122 – 241) and 125 (92 – 170) mmol/l, respectively. LDH and CK did not change significantly over time (Table 1). After reperfusion, lactate levels were significantly higher compared to pre-ischaemia in both groups (p=0.01 and p=0.005 for group C and IPoC, respectively). No differences between the treatment groups were detected.

Table 1: Blood oxidative stress variables during experimental ischaemia

			Control			*IPoC*		
			P	*I*	*R*	*P*	*I*	*R*
Lactate	Absolute	*Median*	1.1	1,9	1,9	1.6	2,15	3,05
		Range	0.8 – 1.4	1,1 - 2,3	1,3 - 2,6	0.9 – 2.2	1 - 3,1	2,1 - 4,2
	Relative	*Median*	100%	168%	217%*	100%	173%	235%**
		Range	-	119 - 360	121 - 414	-	112 - 299	191 - 312
Lactate-dehydrogenase	Absolute	*Median*	151	132	121	147	153	130
		Range	123 – 206	97 - 173	93 - 159	122 – 241	95 - 214	86 - 202
	Relative	*Median*	100%	100%	98%	100%	97%	101%
		Range	-	64 - 147	80 - 120	-	78 - 161	78 - 142
Creatinine-kinase	Absolute	*Median*	122	108	103	125	104	111
		Range	88 – 180	64 - 169	83 - 165	92 – 170	76 - 126	84 - 122
	Relative	*Median*	100%	102%	99%	100%	98%	100%
		Range	-	65 - 124,4	93 - 138	-	70 - 162	85 - 178

Plasma levels of lactate, lactate-dehydrogenase and creatinine-kinase were measured at the different time points (P = pre-ischaemia, I = Ischaemia, R = Reperfusion) in horses belonging to a control group (group C) and a group subjected postconditioning (group IPoC). The values are expressed as absolute value as mmol/l, and as percentage compared to the pre-ischaemia time point. There were no significant differences between the groups. Significant differences within the groups compared to the pre-ischaemia time point are marked with an asterisk (p<0.05; ** p<0.01).*

Discussion

The main finding of this study is that the horses subjected to IPoC exhibited a lower mucosal apoptotic cell count indicated by fewer cleaved caspase 3 positive cells (Fig 1). Moreover, in the control group the cell death progressed during reperfusion with a significant increase of both cleaved-caspase-3 and TUNEL positive cells, which could not be detected in the postconditioned group. This confirms our hypothesis that IPoC decreases apoptosis in the equine intestine after ischaemia/reperfusion injury. The inflammatory cell count (Fig. 2), mucosal HSP-70 staining (Fig 4), blood lactate level (Table 1) and tissue SOD, MDA and MPO levels (Fig 8) were all significantly affected by ischaemia and/or reperfusion. However, no differences between the treatment groups could be detected. Therefore, we rejected the hypotheses that IPoC would decrease inflammation, neuronal cell death and oxidative stress, and that IPoC would be accompanied by an increased heat shock response.

Intestinal IPoC studies in rat models have also demonstrated decreased levels of apoptotic markers in animals subjected to IPoC, reporting lower TUNEL positive cell counts (15-18, 33), and cleaved caspase-3 expression (15, 16). A previous study in horses undergoing IPoC could demonstrate less epithelial denudation and lower paracellular permeability after experimental intestinal ischaemia (30). These positive effects may be explained by the lower apoptosis cell count found in the current analysis, and may indicate a protective effect of IPoC on ischaemia reperfusion injury in horses. A potential mechanism of IPoC may involve the attenuation of apoptosis via the downregulation of PDCD4 and Fas-L (17), or the activation of JAK/STAT pathway (34); however, these pathways were not investigated in the current study.

Intestinal ischaemia leads to hypoxia and concurrent oxidative stress (2). In the investigated variables for oxidative stress, an effect of the experimental segmental ischaemia could be observed in the intestinal tissue analysis (Fig 8). SOD activity was significantly decreased after ischaemia, indicating the presence of reactive oxygen species. Subjectively, the MDA level increased during ischaemia indicating increased lipid peroxidation; however, the only significant change over time was found between the PR sample and ischaemia (group C) or reperfusion (group IPoC). Looking at the blood analysis, only lactate levels were significantly higher during reperfusion (Table 1). Plasma LDH and CK were within reference values during all time points and did not change over time. Contrary to the significant changes in oxidative stress levels found in studies investigating IPoC in a rat model (14-16, 18-20, 33, 35), we found no differences between the treatment groups, contradicting an effect of IPoC on oxidative stress in the applied experimental model. A possible explanation may be that the low flow ischaemia implemented in this study elicited less oxidative stress than the complete occlusion of the cranial mesenteric artery (CMA) performed in the rat model. Regarding the systemic variables for oxidative stress, the intestinal segment subjected to segmental ischaemia may have been too short to elicit significant systemic effects. Moreover, the anaesthetic management of the horses with intravenous fluids and inotropic drugs also may have ameliorated the systemic effect. Smaller differences between the groups may not have been detected due to the relatively high variance between the samples combined with the low sample size. Individual variation between the horses may explain a higher variance compared to the relatively homogenous test population in rodent studies.

The serosa of the reperfusion and PR samples showed similar inflammatory infiltration by the presence of calprotectin positive cells (Fig. 2). In contrast, the mucosa did reveal a difference between these samples, exhibiting more inflammatory cells in the reperfusion sample compared to the PR sample. The inflammatory infiltrate in this proximal segment that has not been subjected to ischaemia, could represent an effect of the laparotomy and concurrent tissue manipulation (36, 37), or may be the result of remote intestinal reperfusion injury. The latter has also been found by other authors, reporting increased neutrophilic infiltration in the proximal resection margins of naturally occurring strangulating obstructions (38, 39). This serosal influx of neutrophils is a normal site of entry into the intestinal wall after reperfusion injury (2, 38, 40, 41). Only group IPoC showed a significantly higher calprotectin cell count in the serosa of the reperfusion and PR samples compared to the pre-ischaemia and ischaemia samples. The prolonged intestinal exteriorisation and manipulation necessary for performing IPoC, could possibly evoke a more pronounced neutrophilic response in the serosa. Another explanation may be that IPoC elicited a more severe inflammatory response due to reperfusion related injury. This could represent a potential disadvantage and a contraindication for performing IPoC in clinical cases. On the other hand, there were no significant differences in a direct comparison between the groups. Therefore, the relevance of these observations is questionable.

As additional marker for inflammation, MPO activity was quantified in the intestinal tissue (Fig 8C), which has been shown to be lower in rats undergoing IPoC (15, 16, 18, 19). This heme-enzyme is predominantly present in neutrophils, but is also expressed in monocytes and macrophages (42, 43). The MPO activity in the intestinal tissue was significantly lower in the proximal intestinal segment compared to the reperfusion segments. Comparing this to the calprotectin positive cell counts, this may reflect the lower cell count in the mucosa of the proximal samples. As with the calprotectin positive cell counts, no difference was found between the groups. This suggests that IPoC does not significantly alter the inflammatory infiltrate in the current model, and that the reduced apoptosis level after IPoC is not mediated through a decreased neutrophilic response.

The neuronal count in the myenteric plexus was not significantly affected by ischaemia or reperfusion (Fig 6), possibly related to a relatively short timeframe of the current study. Studies investigating the effect of experimental small intestinal ischaemia in rodents, have shown that neuronal loss was not apparent before 24 h of reperfusion (44), and that apoptosis of enteric neurons detected by TUNEL stain could not be found before 6 h (32, 45). Evaluating the myenteric plexus in the cleaved-caspase-3 and TUNEL stained intestinal sections, no immunoreactivity of the myenteric plexus was found. A more short term marker of cell damage is the change in the distribution of Hu immunoreactivity towards the nucleus, which has been detected as early as 1 hour post-ischaemia (32). We could not observe any nuclear Hu staining, possibly indicating the duration of reperfusion might not be the only cause for the absence of detectable ischaemia reperfusion injury to the enteric neurons. The application of different ischaemia models could also account for this disparity. Nitrergic neurons have been reported to account for 23–52% of all myenteric neurons in rodents (9, 31), with an increased NOS ratio after 48 h of reperfusion in response to ischaemia (32). The basal NOS ratio in the current study was slightly lower at 21-22%, without any changes after ischaemia or reperfusion. The submucosal neuronal plexus may have responded differently; however, this was not investigated in the current study.

The highly stress-inducible HSP-70 has been shown to guide co-translational folding for protein maturation and to restore folding after injury, thereby promoting cell survival (46). This is the first report of the heat shock response in experimental equine small intestinal ischaemia. Pre-ischaemia, HSP-70 was predominantly located in the cytoplasm, and exhibited an increase in nuclear immunoreactivity during reperfusion (Fig 4). This nuclear shift has been reported in clinical cases of acute intestinal ischaemia in humans and horses (47, 48). Cell culture experiments have found that HSP-70 translocates to the nucleus during cellular stress, and relocates to the cytoplasm as the cell recovers (49, 50). This is considered as part of the stress response and possibly promotes cell survival by maintaining or restoring the epigenetic regulating proteins in the nucleus (46, 50, 51). In the equine study, increased HSP-70 immunoreactivity of the intestinal segment proximal to the strangulating obstruction was not related to the clinical outcome (47). Several studies investigating ischaemic preconditioning in laboratory animals, have implicated that increased inducible HSP-70 expression contributes to the protective mechanism of preconditioning (27-29, 52). However, we could not detect an effect of IPoC on the expression or distribution of this protein.

Limitations of the current study are the small sample size and high variance in some of the data sets, possibly precluding the detection of smaller differences. Furthermore, there was no direct comparison with reperfusion injury. As mentioned previously, the duration of ischaemia and reperfusion may have been too short for complete evaluation of some of the tested variables. Moreover, the long-term effect of IPoC could not be assessed. The duration of the experimental ischaemia and reperfusion was limited, because extended anaesthesia times in horses can compromise cardiovascular stability and induce muscular damage and inflammation. Letting the horses recover from anaesthesia prior to euthanasia was considered unethical. Pharmacological preconditioning with xylazine and isoflurane administered for anaesthetic premedication and maintenance, may have mitigated the potential effect of the ischaemic injury or IPoC. However, this effect was present in both groups. A limitation of the TUNEL assay is that it may identify both apoptotic and necrotic cells by labelling double stranded DNA breaks that are produced during early necrosis (53-55), complicating the interpretation of the results. Cleaved caspase-3 is specific for apoptosis, yet this effector caspase does not indicate through which pathway the apoptosis was initiated (56). Therefore, the quantification of early initiator caspases or markers for cell necrosis could have provided more clarity on the mechanism of cell death. Another limitation, is that the difference in ischaemia model precludes the direct comparison with previous reports investigating IPoC in a rat model. Nevertheless, the segmental jejunal ischaemia model is more representative for clinical strangulating colic in horses. The CMA model is used as a model for human intestinal ischaemia, which is suitable for the more generalized obstruction of the cranial mesenteric artery described in humans (57). For clinical cases with local strangulating obstructions such as small bowel volvulus and incarcerating hernias, the current animal model may be more appropriate (58).

Conclusion

Fewer apoptotic cells were found in the mucosa of the horses subjected to IPoC. This could indicate a protective effect on small intestinal ischaemia reperfusion injury in horses, yet this cannot be concluded without direct comparison with histomorphological injury. None of the other tested variables were significantly affected by IPoC, suggesting only a limited impact. These negative results are in contradiction with the findings of many rodent studies investigating IPoC in small intestinal ischaemia. This disparity may be caused by a difference in species, anaesthetic protocol, the applied ischaemia model and the degree of ischaemic injury. Therefore, further research on the mechanism of action of IPoC in equine segmental ischaemia and its effect in clinical cases of strangulating colic is needed. Although not significantly affected by IPoC, the observed increase in nuclear HSP-70 after reperfusion suggests that this molecular chaperone may be of relevance in the equine intestinal response to ischaemia, warranting further investigation.

Materials and Methods

Experimental design

The study was reviewed by the Ethics Committee for Animal Experiments of Lower Saxony, Germany, and approved according to §8 of the German Animal Welfare Act (LAVES 33.8-42502-04-18/2856). A power analysis was performed prior to commencing the study using free available software (G*Power 3.1.9.2, Heinrich Heine Universität, Düsseldorf, Germany). To detect a difference of 25 cells/mm2 in the immunohistochemistry cell counts with a standard deviation of 15 cells/mm2, a sample size of 7 horses per treatment group was required, based on a power of 0.8 and alpha of 0.05. Fourteen horses, owned by the university, were assigned to a group subjected to ischaemic postconditioning (group IPoC; n=7) and a control group (group C, n=7) using simple randomisation with an equal allocation ratio.

Animals

Group C consisted of five Warmbloods, one Islandic horse and one Thoroughbred, with a mean age of 12.6 ± 8.7 years and mean weight of 535 ± 89 kg. Group IPoC consisted of four Warmbloods, one Islandic pony, one Thoroughbred, and one Standardbred, with a mean age of 10.4 ± 8.6 years and weight of 506 ± 96 kg. All horses were systemically healthy, and had been elected for euthanasia due to severe orthopaedic problems. Faecal egg counts were done, and all were below the cut-off value of 200 eggs per gram. The horses were stabled at the facilities of the equine clinic at least two weeks prior to surgery. No medication was administered during this time. The horses had free access to hay and water and were hand walked daily. Prior to anaesthesia, feed but not water was withheld for 6 hours.

Anaesthesia and surgical procedure

After premedication with 0.7 mg/kg body weight (BW) xylazine (Xylavet 20 mg/ml, CP-Pharma GmbH, Burgdorf, Germany), general anaesthesia was induced with 0.1 mg/kg BW diazepam (Ziapam 5 mg/kg, Ecuphar GmbH, Greifswald, Germany) and 2.2 mg/kg ketamine (Narketan,

Vétoquinol GmbH, Ismaning, Germany). Anaesthesia was maintained with isoflurane (Isofluran CP, CP-Pharma GmbH) in 100% oxygen, and continuous rate infusions with lactated Ringer's solution (Ringer-Laktat EcobagClick, B. Braun Melsungen AG, Melsungen, Germany) and dobutamine (Dobutamin-ratiopharm 250mg, Ratiopharm GmbH, Ulm, Germany) were given to effect, to maintain the mean arterial blood pressure between 60 and 80 mmHg. A routine pre-umbilical median laparotomy was performed in dorsal recumbency. Segmental small intestinal ischaemia was induced in 1.5 m jejunum by occlusion of the mesenteric arteries and veins with umbilical tape. The ligature was tightened under monitoring of the intestinal microperfusion with microlightguide spectophotometry and laser Doppler fluxmetry (O2C, LEA Medizintechnik GmbH, Giessen, Germany), and the ligature was tied as soon as the blood flow was reduced by 90%. The ischaemia was maintained for 90 min. In between the different stages of the experiment, the intestines were replaced in the abdominal cavity and the laparotomy was temporarily closed with towel clamps. In group C, the ligature was released without manipulation of the vessels or the intestine. In group IPoC, postconditioning was implemented after release of ischaemia by clamping the mesenteric vessels with large haemostatic forceps, with the jaws covered with latex catheters to decrease trauma to the vessel walls. This elicited complete vascular occlusion as confirmed by laser Doppler Fluxmetry. Clamping was performed for 3 cycles of 30 sec, alternated with 30 sec of reperfusion, which is the most commonly reported intestinal IPoC algorithm (16-18, 21, 59). Following ischaemia, a reperfusion duration of 120 minutes was implemented in both groups. Subsequently, the horses were euthanized by intravenous administration of 90 mg/kg pentobarbital (Release 50 mg/ml, WDT eG, Garbsen, Germany) without regaining consciousness. Everyone involved in the experimental trial was aware of the group allocation of the horses during the conduct of the experiment.

Sample collection

Full thickness intestinal segments of 10 cm jejunum were taken just before induction of ischaemia (pre-ischaemia sample, P), at the end of ischaemia (ischaemia sample, I), and at the end of reperfusion (reperfusion sample, R). At this time point, an additional intestinal sample was taken from the segment just proximal (orad) to the post-ischaemic segment (proximal sample, PR). The lumen of the remaining intestinal segments was occluded with umbilical tape and lavaged prior to replacement in the abdominal cavity. Two antimesenterial sections of 2 cm2 from each sample were fixed in a 4% formaldehyde solution and subsequently embedded in paraffin following standard procedure. Smaller sections of full thickness tissue from the antimesenterial intestine were snap frozen in liquid nitrogen, and stored at -80 °C until further processing. Blood samples were taken from the jugular vein and the facial artery at the end of the pre-ischaemic, ischaemic, and reperfusion periods and collected in heparinised tubes.

Immunohistochemistry

To quantify the number of apoptotic and necrotic cells, paraffin sections were immunohistochemically stained for cleaved-caspase-3 (dilution 1:200, rabbit-anti-human, CleavedCaspase-3Asp175 antibody, Cell Signalling Technology Europe B.V., Leiden, The Netherlands), and terminal deoxynucleotidyl transferase dUTP nick end labelling (TUNEL) (ApopTag® Peroxidase In Situ Apoptosis Detection Kit, Merck KGaA, Darmstadt, Germany) was performed as described previously (60). Furthermore, sections were stained for cytosolic calprotectin using monoclonal mouse anti-human myeloid/histiocyte antigen (clone MAC 387, DakoCytomation, Glostrup, Denmark) as described elsewhere (61). Immunohistochemical staining for HSP-70 was also performed. In short, the slides were demasked by heating in citrate solution, followed by blocking with 20 % goat serum. The slides were incubated overnight with 1:400 polyclonal rabbit antibody against inducible HSP-70 (Anti-Hsp70 antibody ab79852, Abcam, Cambridge, UK), followed by incubation with secondary antibody (1:200 goat-anti-rabbit) and then the ABC reagent (Vectastain ABC, Biozol diagnostics Vertrieb GmbH, Eching, Germany). The negative control was incubated with 1:2000 rabbit serum (R4505, Sigma Aldrich Merck KGaA, Darmstadt, Germany) instead of the primary antibody. Equine testicular tissue was used as a positive control. Further processing was performed with the same protocol as described for the other stainings.

All slides were scanned to a digital format at 20x magnification (Axio Scan.Z1, Carl Zeiss GmbH, Oberkochen, Germany), and subsequently evaluated using the accompanying software (Zen Blue 3.0, Carl Zeiss GmbH). One section per sample was evaluated by one observer (NV trained by MHT and CP), who was blinded to the identity of the slides. For the cleaved-caspase-3 and TUNEL stained slides, the positive cell count in the mucosa was determined. The calprotectin positive cells were counted separately in the mucosa, submucosa, muscularis and serosa. The surface area of a section of 10 to 15 villi was determined in mm2. Following manual counting of the positive cells, the cell counts were expressed in cells/mm2.

Due to the more diffuse staining pattern in the HSP-70 stained slides, a semi-quantitative score for enterocyte immunoreactivity was developed. The enterocyte cytoplasm and nuclei were graded separately for staining intensity (0 – absent to very weak, 1 – low, 2 - moderate, 3 – intense) in the crypts, the villus base and villus apex, at a standard fixed colour setting for all sections. For further analysis, the cytoplasm scores (0-3) were added up, resulting in a total mucosa cytoplasm score (0-9) per section, and the same was done for the nucleus scores. The muscularis propria was given one grade for its cytoplasmic staining intensity. The nuclei in the muscularis were not scored separately, since these exhibited a similar staining intensity throughout all the sections.

In 7 horses (3 in group C, 4 in group IPoC), additional immunohistochemical staining for Hu and nitric oxide synthase (NOS) was performed to evaluate the number, proportion and morphology of the neurons in the jejunal myenteric plexus in samples P, I and R. The full thickness intestinal tissue was fixed in a solution containing 4% paraformaldehyde and 0.002% picric acid in 0.1 mol/l phosphate buffer overnight at 4°C. Subsequently, a whole mount preparation of the myenteric plexus was performed removing the different intestinal layers by careful manual dissection. Then the tissue was incubated for 1 h in phosphate buffered saline (PBS)/NaN3 (0.1 %)/horse serum (HS, 4%) (Sigma Aldrich, Darmstadt, Germany) to avoid unspecific staining. After this, the tissue was incubated 48 h with the primary antibodies (Mouse α Hu-Biotin 1:50, Alexis, San Diego, USA; Rabbit α NOS 1:3000, Molecular Probes, Eugene, USA). Subsequently, the tissue was washed (3 x 10 min) in phosphate buffer and then incubated for 12 h with the secondary antibodies (Donkey α rabbit Cy2 1:200, Streptavidin Cy3 1:500, Jackson ImmunoResearch, Cambridgeshire, United Kingdom). Finally, specimens were washed in PBS, mounted on poly-l-lysine-coated slides and cover slipped with a solution of PBS (pH 7.0) /NaN3 (0.1) containing 65% glycerol. The preparations were examined with an epifluorescence microscope (Olympus IX70, Olympus, Hamburg, Germany), equipped with appropriate filter blocks. Images were acquired and analysed with a monochrome camera (XM 10; Olympus) using the Olympus cellSens standard software. The neuronal count was performed in a blinded manner. Neurons were counted in 50 ganglia per sample. The neuronal counts of the individual horses were grouped based on the time point and test group. To adjust for the high variability between the horses, relative cell counts of the ischaemia and reperfusion sample were determined per horse as the percentage of the pre-ischaemia sample mean. Furthermore, the percentage of NOS immunoreactive neurons compared to the total neuron (Hu) count was determined.

Enzymatic assays

The full thickness intestinal tissue was homogenised in assay specific lysis buffers as described below using a high-speed homogenisator (FastPrep-24™ 5G, MP Biomedicals Germany GmbH, Eschwege, Germany). Protein content of each individual homogenized sample was assessed by performing a Bradford assay, as described previously (62).

The SOD activity was detected using a commercially available colorimetric assay kit (19160 SOD Determination Kit, Sigma Aldrich/Merck KGaA) after homogenisation in an appropriate lysis buffer (CB cell lysis buffer, Cell Biologics, Chicago, USA). The SOD activity assay relies on the formation of formazin dye (absorbance at 450 nm), when tetrazolium salt is reduced with a superoxide anion. Bovine SOD (Superoxide Dismutase Bovine Erythrocytes, Merck KGaA) was used to establish a concentration curve. MPO activity was determined based on its ability to catalyse the formation of hypochlorous acid using a commercially available assay kit, which included lysis buffer and positive controls (Myeloperoxidase Colorimetric Activity Assay Kit, Sigma Aldrich/Merck KGaA). The MDA content was determined by measuring the colorimetric (532 nm) product that forms when MDA reacts with thiobarbituric acid, with an assay kit including lysis buffer and positive controls (Lipid Peroxidation Assay Kit, Sigma Aldrich/Merck KGaA). The kits were used in accordance with manufacturer's instructions, with only a small modification in the MDA assay. Here, butanol (1:2 of total volume) was added for the purification of the samples, and the colorimetric measurements were performed on the organic layer, without prior evaporation of the butanol.

All assays were analysed using a microplate spectrophotometer (Epoch, Biotek Germany, Bad Friedrichshall, Germany). To correct for the variation in protein content between the individual samples after homogenisation, all values were expressed as units (SOD or MPO activity) or nMol (MDA levels) per mg protein in the sample. The assays were performed in duplicates and the mean of both values was used for further analysis. Concentration curves were plotted by use of commercially available software (Graphpad Prism 8.4.2, Graphpad Software Inc., San Diego, California, USA), and a r2 value of >0.97 was considered appropriate. In the MPO measurements the negative values close to zero, were set to zero to enable statistical analysis.

Blood analysis

LDH and CK were measured in plasma immediately after sampling by use of a commercially available analyser (cobas c311, Roche/Hitachi, Mannheim, Germany). Arterial blood samples for lactate measurement were taken at the same time and analysed immediately (ABL825 flex, Radiometer Medical ApS, Bronshoj, Denmark). For comparison between the time points and groups, a correction for haemodilution was made by measuring albumin in the corresponding samples and expressing the values as mmol/g albumin. Subsequently, the ischaemia and reperfusion samples were expressed as relative values compared to pre-ischaemia.

Data Analysis

Statistical analysis and graph design were performed using commercial software (Graphpad Prism 8.4.2, Graphpad Software Inc., San Diego, California, USA). Normal distribution was assessed with the Shapiro Wilks test and by visual inspection of QQ plots of the model residuals. The normal distributed data were expressed as mean (± SD), and data that did not show normal or lognormal distribution, were expressed as median (min-max). The equality of variances was tested by visual assessment of the homoscedasticity plots, and by performing Levene's test. Statistical significance was set at $p<0.05$.

For analysis of the normally distributed data, a two-way repeated measures ANOVA was performed for one independent effect (group), and the time points as repeated effect. This was implemented to compare the values between the different time points and groups, with the horses as subject effect. The Geisser-Greenhouse correction was applied for the p-values. Multiple pairwise comparisons were performed with a post-hoc Tukey test to compare the different time points within the groups, and a post-hoc Sidak test for group comparison.

For the normally distributed SOD and MDA results, the ROUT outlier test was implemented with the maximum desired False Discovery Rate (Q) set at 1%. After testing for equality of variance, mixed effect model fitted as a two-way repeated measures ANOVA for missing values was performed for one independent effect (group), and the time points as repeated effect. Post hoc testing was performed as described above.

For the ordinal and not normally distributed data (HSP-score, MPO units), distribution free nonparametric models were used for independent (treatment and control group) and correlated (time points) effects. A Mann-Whitney-U test was executed to compare the results between the different groups at each time point. For comparing the correlated different time points, a Friedman test in combination with the post hoc Dunns-test for multiple pairwise comparisons were performed.

Declarations

Acknowledgements

The authors would like to thank Doris Voigtländer and Marion Langeheine from the Institute for Anatomy, Kerstin Rohn from the Institute of Pathology and Susanne Hoppe from the Institute of Physiology and Cell Biology for their expert support in tissue processing and immunohistochemistry. We are very grateful for the technical support we received from Silke Akhdar from the Department of Biochemistry in the execution of the enzyme assays. We would also like to thank all involved employees of the Clinic for Horses who contributed to the care of the horses or who gave their support in the execution of the study.

Authors' contributions

All authors contributed to the manuscript. NV contributed to the study design and execution, and performed the data analysis and interpretation. NB, MKB, MHT, CP, GMW and SK contributed to the study design as well as the data analysis and interpretation. HS contributed to the study execution and data analysis. The author(s) read and approved the final manuscript.

Funding

This study was funded by a research grant from the European College of Veterinary Surgeons (2019 LA, NV) and by a research grant from Stiftung ProPferd (2019/04, SK/NV). This project was partially supported by Zoonosenplattform with the BMBF/DLR project HypoxiaInfect (MKB). This publication was supported by Deutsche Forschungsgemeinschaft and University of Veterinary Medicine Hannover, Foundation within the funding program Open Access Publishing. The funders had no role in study design, data collection and analysis, decision to publish, or preparation of the manuscript. Open Access funding enabled and organized by Projekt DEAL.

Availability of data and materials

The datasets analysed in the current study are available in the Mendeley repository, openly available under the following reference: Verhaar, Nicole (2020), "Ischaemic Postconditioning in Equine Jejunal Ischaemia" MendeleyData, doi.org/10.17632/mxhhxpvpvj.2

Ethics approval and consent to participate

The study including all experimental protocols was reviewed by the Ethics Committee for Animal Experiments of Lower Saxony, Germany, and approved according to §8 of the German Animal Welfare Act (LAVES 33.8–42,502–04-18/2856). All methods were carried out in accordance with relevant guidelines and regulations. The study was carried out in compliance with the ARRIVE guidelines.

Consent for publication - Not applicable.

Competing interests - the authors declare that they have no competing interests.

References

(1) Auer JA, Stick JA, Kuemmerle JM, Prange T. Equine Surgery. 5th ed: Elsevier Health Sciences, St. Louis, Missouri; 2019.

(2) Blikslager AT. The Equine Acute Abdomen: John Wiley & Sons, Hoboken, New Jersey; 2017.

(3) Park P, Haglund U, Bulkley G, Fält K. The sequence of development of intestinal tissue injury after strangulation ischemia and reperfusion. Surgery. 1990;107(5):574-80.

(4) Lundin C, Sullins K, White N, Clem M, Debowes R, Pfeiffer C. Induction of peritoneal adhesions with small intestinal ischaemia and distention in the foal. Equine veterinary journal. 1989;21(6):451-8.

(5) Laws EG, Freeman DE. Significance of reperfusion injury after venous strangulation obstruction of equine jejunum. Journal of Investigative Surgery. 1995;8(4):263-70.

(6) Prichard M, Ducharme NG, Wilkins PA, Erb HN, Butt M. Xanthine oxidase formation during experimental ischemia of the equine small intestine. Canadian Journal of Veterinary Research. 1991;55(4):310.

(7) Vatistas NJ, Snyder JR, Hildebrand S, Harmon FA, Woliner MJ, Barry SJ, et al. Effects of U-74389G, a novel 21-aminosteroid, on small intestinal ischemia and reperfusion injury in horses. American journal of veterinary research. 1996;57(5):762-70.

(8) Türler A, Kalff JC, Moore BA, Hoffman RA, Billiar TR, Simmons RL, et al. Leukocyte-derived inducible nitric oxide synthase mediates murine postoperative ileus. Annals of surgery. 2006;244(2):220.

(9) Bodi N, Szalai Z, Bagyanszki M. Nitrergic Enteric Neurons in Health and Disease-Focus on Animal Models. Int J Mol Sci. 2019;20(8).

(10) Krenz M, Baines C, Kalogeris T, Korthuis R, editors. Cell survival programs and ischemia/reperfusion: hormesis, preconditioning, and cardioprotection. Colloquium Series on Integrated Systems Physiology: From Molecule to Function to Disease; Morgan & Claypool Life Sciences, Williston, Vermont; 2013.

(11) Zhi-Qing Zhao JSC, Michael E. Halkos, Faraz Kerendi,, Ning-Ping Wang RAG, and Jakob Vinten-Johansen. Inhibition of myocardial injury by ischemic postconditioning during reperfusion: comparison with ischemic preconditioning. Am J Physiol Heart Circ Physiol. 2003;285:579-88.

(12) Feyzizadeh S, Badalzadeh R. Application of ischemic postconditioning's algorithms in tissues protection: response to methodological gaps in preclinical and clinical studies. J Cell Mol Med. 2017;21(10):2257-67.

(13) Santos CHMd, Dourado DM, Sampaio TL, Dias LdES, Almeida MHMd, Oliva JVDG, et al. Effect of postconditioning and atorvastatin in preventing remote intestinal reperfusion injury. J Coloproctology. 2017;37(4):301-5.

(14) Liu KX, Li YS, Huang WQ, Chen SQ, Wang ZX, Liu JX, et al. Immediate postconditioning during reperfusion attenuates intestinal injury. Intensive Care Med. 2009;35(5):933-42.

(15) Cheng C-H, Lin H-C, Lai IR, Lai H-S. Ischemic postconditioning attenuate reperfusion injury of small intestine: impact of mitochondrial permeability transition. Transplantation. 2013;95(4):559-65.

(16) Wen SH, Ling YH, Li Y, Li C, Liu JX, Li YS, et al. Ischemic postconditioning during reperfusion attenuates oxidative stress and intestinal mucosal apoptosis induced by intestinal ischemia/reperfusion via aldose reductase. Surgery. 2013;153(4):555-64.

(17) Jia Z, Lian W, Shi H, Cao C, Han S, Wang K, et al. Ischemic Postconditioning Protects Against Intestinal Ischemia/Reperfusion Injury via the HIF-1alpha/miR-21 Axis. Sci Rep. 2017;7(1):16190.

(18) Weiwei Chu SL, Shanwei Wang, Aili Yan, Lei Nie. Ischemic postconditioning provides protection against ischemia-reperfusion injury in intestines of rats. Int J Clin Exp Pathol. 2015;8(6):6474 - 81.

(19) Sengul I, Sengul D, Guler O, Hasanoglu A, Urhan MK, Taner AS, et al. Postconditioning attenuates acute intestinal ischemia-reperfusion injury. Kaohsiung J Med Sci. 2013;29(3):119-27.

(20) Rosero O, Onody P, Stangl R, Turoczi Z, Fulop A, Garbaisz D, et al. Postconditioning of the small intestine: which is the most effective algorithm in a rat model? J Surg Res. 2014;187(2):427-37.

(21) Li YS, Wang ZX, Li C, Xu M, Li Y, Huang WQ, et al. Proteomics of ischemia/reperfusion injury in rat intestine with and without ischemic postconditioning. J Surg Res. 2010;164(1):e173-80.

(22) Buchholz B, Donato M, D'Annunzio V, Gelpi RJ. Ischemic postconditioning: mechanisms, comorbidities, and clinical application. Molecular and cellular biochemistry. 2014;392(1-2):1-12.

(23) Whitley D, Goldberg SP, Jordan WD. Heat shock proteins: a review of the molecular chaperones. J Vasc Surg. 1999;29(4):748-51.

(24) Oksala NK, Kaarniranta K, Tenhunen JJ, Tiihonen R, Heino A, Sistonen L, et al. Reperfusion but not acute ischemia in pig small intestine induces transcriptionally mediated heat shock response in situ. Eur Surg Res. 2002;34(6):397-404.

(25) Fleming SD, Starnes BW, Kiang JG, Stojadinovic A, Tsokos GC, Shea-Donohue T. Heat stress protection against mesenteric I/R-induced alterations in intestinal mucosa in rats. J Appl Physiol (1985). 2002;92(6):2600-7.

(26) Tons C, Klosterhalfen B, Klein HM, Rau HM, Anurov M, Oettinger A, et al. Induction of heat shock protein 70 (HSP70) by zinc bis (DL-hydrogen aspartate) reduces ischemic small-bowel tissue damage in rats. Langenbecks Arch Chir. 1997;382(1):43-8.

(27) Yin C, Salloum FN, Kukreja RC. A novel role of microRNA in late preconditioning: upregulation of endothelial nitric oxide synthase and heat shock protein 70. Circ Res. 2009;104(5):572-5.

(28) Sun X-C, Xian X-H, Li W-B, Li L, Yan C-Z, Li Q-J, et al. Activation of p38 MAPK participates in brain ischemic tolerance induced by limb ischemic preconditioning by up-regulating HSP 70. Exp Neurology. 2010;224(2):347-55.

(29) Selimoglu O, Ugurlucan M, Basaran M, Gungor F, Banach M, Cucu O, et al. Efficacy of remote ischaemic preconditioning for spinal cord protection against ischaemic injury: association with heat shock protein expression. Folia Neuropathol. 2008;46(3):204-12.

(30) Verhaar N, Breves G, Hewicker-Trautwein M, Pfarrer C, Rohn K, Burmester M, et al. The effect of ischaemic postconditioning on mucosal integrity and function in equine jejunal ischaemia. Equine Vet J. 2021;00:1-11

(31) Qu Z-D, Thacker M, Castelucci P, Bagyanszki M, Epstein ML, Furness JB. Immunohistochemical analysis of neuron types in the mouse small intestine. Cell and tissue research. 2008;334(2):147-61.

(32) Rivera LR, Thacker M, Pontell L, Cho H-J, Furness JB. Deleterious effects of intestinal ischemia/reperfusion injury in the mouse enteric nervous system are associated with protein nitrosylation. Cell and tissue research. 2011;344(1):111-23.

(33) Yang M, Dong J-X, Li L-B, Che H-J, Yong J, Song F-B, et al. Local and remote postconditioning decrease intestinal injury in a rabbit ischemia/reperfusion model. Gastroenterology Research and Practice. 2016;2016.

(34) Wen SH, Li Y, Li C, Xia ZQ, Liu WF, Zhang XY, et al. Ischemic postconditioning during reperfusion attenuates intestinal injury and mucosal cell apoptosis by inhibiting JAK/STAT signaling activation. Shock. 2012;38(4):411-9.

(35) Chen R, Zhang Y-y, Lan J-n, Liu H-m, Li W, Wu Y, et al. Ischemic Postconditioning Alleviates Intestinal Ischemia-Reperfusion Injury by Enhancing Autophagy and Suppressing Oxidative Stress through the Akt/GSK-3β/Nrf2 Pathway in Mice. Oxidative Medicine and Cellular Longevity. 2020;2020.

(36) Bauck AG, Grosche A, Morton AJG, Vickroy TW, Freeman DE. Effect of lidocaine on in ammation in equine jejunum subjected to manipulation only and remote to intestinal segments subjected to ischemia. AJVR. 2017;78(8):977 - 89.

(37) Hopster-Iversen CC, Hopster K, Staszyk C, Rohn K, Freeman DE, Rötting AK. Effects of experimental mechanical manipulations on local inflammation in the jejunum of horses. Am J Vet Res. 2014;75(4):385-91.

(38) Little D, Tomlinson JE, Blikslager AT. Post operative neutrophilic inflammation in equine small intestine after manipulation and ischaemia. Equine Vet J. 2005;37(4):329-35.

(39) Gerard M, Blikslager A, Roberts M, Tate Jr L, Argenzio R. The characteristics of intestinal injury peripheral to strangulating obstruction lesions in the equine small intestine. Equine veterinary journal. 1999;31(4):331-5.

(40) Dabareiner RM, Sullins KE, Snyder JR, White NA, 2nd, Gardner IA. Evaluation of the microcirculation of the equine small intestine after intraluminal distention and subsequent decompression. Am J Vet Res. 1993;54(10):1673-82.

(41) Dabareiner RM, Snyder JR, Sullins KE, White NA, 2nd, Gardner IA. Evaluation of the microcirculation of the equine jejunum and ascending colon after ischemia and reperfusion. Am J Vet Res. 1993;54(10):1683-92.

(42) Sugiyama S, Okada Y, Sukhova GK, Virmani R, Heinecke JW, Libby P. Macrophage myeloperoxidase regulation by granulocyte macrophage colony-stimulating factor in human atherosclerosis and implications in acute coronary syndromes. The American journal of pathology. 2001;158(3):879-91.

(43) Bos A, Wever R, Roos D. Characterization and quantification of the peroxidase in human monocytes. Biochimica et Biophysica Acta (BBA)-Enzymology. 1978;525(1):37-44.

(44) Lindeström L-M, Ekblad E. Structural and neuronal changes in rat ileum after ischemia with reperfusion. Digestive diseases and sciences. 2004;49(7-8):1212-22.

(45) Mei F, Guo S, He YT, Zhu J, Zhou DS, Niu JQ, et al. Apoptosis of interstitial cells of Cajal, smooth muscle cells, and enteric neurons induced by intestinal ischemia and reperfusion injury in adult guinea pigs. Virchows Arch. 2009;454(4):401-9.

(46) Welch WJ. Mammalian stress response: cell physiology, structure/function of stress proteins, and implications for medicine and disease. Physiological reviews. 1992;72(4):1063-81.

(47) De Ceulaer K, Delesalle C, Van Elzen R, Van Brantegem L, Weyns A, Van Ginneken C. Morphological data indicate a stress response at the oral border of strangulated small intestine in horses. Res Vet Sci. 2011;91(2):294-300.

(48) Lu XP, Omar RA, Chang WW. Immunocytochemical expression of the 70 kD heat shock protein in ischaemic bowel disease. The Journal of pathology. 1996;179(4):409-13.

(49) Welch WJ, Feramisco J. Nuclear and nucleolar localization of the 72,000-dalton heat shock protein in heat-shocked mammalian cells. Journal of Biological Chemistry. 1984;259(7):4501-13.

(50) Yanoma T, Ogata K, Yokobori T, Ide M, Mochiki E, Toyomasu Y, et al. Heat shock-induced HIKESHI protects cell viability via nuclear translocation of heat shock protein 70. Oncology reports. 2017;38(3):1500-6.

(51) Azkanaz M, Rodríguez López A, de Boer B, Huiting W, Angrand PO, Vellenga E, et al. Protein quality control in the nucleolus safeguards recovery of epigenetic regulators after heat shock. Elife. 2019;8.

(52) Kume M, Yamamoto Y, Saad S, Gomi T, Kimoto S, Shimabukuro T, et al. Ischemic preconditioning of the liver in rats: implications of heat shock protein induction to increase tolerance of ischemia-reperfusion injury. Journal of Laboratory and Clinical Medicine. 1996;128(3):251-8.

(53) Al-Lamki R, Skepper J, Loke Y, King A, Burton G. Apoptosis in the early human placental bed and its discrimination from necrosis using the in-situ DNA ligation technique. Human reproduction (Oxford, England). 1998;13(12):3511-9.

(54) Gold R, Schmied M, Giegerich G, Breitschopf H, Hartung H, Toyka K, et al. Differentiation between cellular apoptosis and necrosis by the combined use of in situ tailing and nick translation techniques. Laboratory investigation; a journal of technical methods and pathology. 1994;71(2):219-25.

(55) Didenko VV, Ngo H, Baskin DS. Early necrotic DNA degradation: presence of blunt-ended DNA breaks, 3' and 5' overhangs in apoptosis, but only 5' overhangs in early necrosis. The American journal of pathology. 2003;162(5):1571-8.

(56) Nuñez G, Benedict MA, Hu Y, Inohara N. Caspases: the proteases of the apoptotic pathway. Oncogene. 1998;17(25):3237-45.

(57) Byard RW. Acute mesenteric ischaemia and unexpected death. Journal of Forensic and Legal Medicine. 2012;19(4):185-90.

(58) Markogiannakis H, Messaris E, Dardamanis D, Pararas N, Tzertzemelis D, Giannopoulos P, et al. Acute mechanical bowel obstruction: clinical presentation, etiology, management and outcome. World journal of gastroenterology: WJG. 2007;13(3):432.

(59) Ferencz A, Takacs I, Horvath S, Ferencz S, Javor S, Fekecs T, et al. Examination of protective effect of ischemic postconditioning after small bowel autotransplantation. Transplant Proc. 2010;42(6):2287-9.

(60) Verhaar N, Pfarrer C, Neudeck S, Konig K, Rohn K, Twele L, et al. Preconditioning with lidocaine and xylazine in experimental equine jejunal ischaemia. Equine Vet J. 2021;53(1):125-133.

(61) Wagner A, Junginger J, Lemensieck F, Hewicker-Trautwein M. Immunohistochemical characterization of gastrointestinal macrophages/phagocytes in dogs with inflammatory bowel disease (IBD) and non-IBD dogs. Veterinary immunology and immunopathology. 2018;197:49-57.

(62) Bradford MM. A rapid and sensitive method for the quantitation of microgram quantities of protein utilizing the principle of protein-dye binding. Analytical biochemistry. 1976;72(1-2):248-54.

8. Manuscript IV

Hypoxia Inducible Factor 1-alpha and 2-alpha distribution during experimental ischaemia of the equine small intestine

Nicole Verhaar[1], Marion Hewicker-Trautwein[2], Christiane Pfarrer[3], Sabine Kästner[1,4]

[1] Clinic for Horses, University of Veterinary Medicine Hannover, Germany

[2] Institute of Pathology, University of Veterinary Medicine Hannover, Germany

[3] Institute for Anatomy, University of Veterinary Medicine Hannover, Germany

[4] Small Animal Clinic, University of Veterinary Medicine Hannover, Germany

Author contribution

- NV contributed to the study design and execution, including the establishment of the immunohistochemical protocols and the microscopic score. NV performed the data analysis and interpretation, and prepared the manuscript.
- MHT, CP, and SK contributed to the study design as well as the data interpretation.
- All authors proofread the manuscript

Summary

Hypoxia inducible factors (HIF) are widely researched as part of hypoxia signalling for their role in different disease processes in human medicine. The objective of this study was to investigate the distribution of these transcription factors in experimental small intestinal ischaemia in the horse.

In 14 horses under general anaesthesia, segmental jejunal ischaemia with 90% reduction in blood flow was implemented. The horses were evenly and randomly divided over two groups, one subjected to ischaemic postconditioning (IPoC) after reperfusion, and a control group undergoing undelayed reperfusion. Intestinal samples were taken pre-ischaemia, after ischaemia and after reperfusion. Immunohistochemical staining for HIF-1α and -2α was performed, and the immunoreactivity pattern in the small intestine was evaluated by light microscopy. The mucosal enterocyte and muscularis staining was recorded for each section using a semi-quantitative score. Comparison between the groups was performed using a Mann-Whitney test, and time points were compared using a Friedman test ($p<0.05$).

No differences between the treatment groups could be detected. For HIF-1α, the reperfusion samples had a significantly higher score in crypt and villus cytoplasmic staining as well as the villus nuclear staining. The score for perinuclear granules in the crypts was significantly lower after reperfusion compared to pre-ischaemia. In HIF-2α stained slides, no nuclear staining was observed, and no significant change in immunoreactivity could be noted over time. A remarkable finding was that 3/14 horses exhibited a distinct intense perinuclear staining pattern in nearly all enterocytes throughout all samples. The other horses demonstrated perinuclear staining in only a small proportion of the enterocytes.

In conclusion, the changes in HIF-1α immunoreactivity over time suggest that this transcription factor plays a role in the intestinal response to ischaemia. HIF-2α did not show any progression during ischaemia or reperfusion. A perinuclear focal HIF-2α staining pattern was associated with individual horses and not with time points, requiring further investigation. We could not detect a difference in HIF-1α and -2α immunoreactivity between the treatment groups, possibly indicating that these factors are not of relevance for postconditioning in the current experimental model. However, this is based on a semi-quantitative score, and a quantitative analysis may be more sensitive.

Introduction

It has been shown that most transcriptional responses to hypoxia are mediated by hypoxia-inducible factors (HIF) (1, 2). HIF-1α expression increases in ischaemic intestinal mucosa (3), and HIF-1α dependent regulation of claudin-1 plays an important role in intestinal epithelial tight junction integrity (4). It has been suggested that the duration and severity of the ischaemia-reperfusion (I/R) insult dictate whether HIF-1 plays a deleterious or protective role (5). Moreover, several authors have found an association between HIF-1α levels and the extent of tissue injury in different experimental models (6-8). Hence it remains unclear if the magnitude of the HIF-1α response is a marker for the protective response, for the degree of I/R injury, or both. The expression of the isoform HIF-2α has also been shown to increase in different tissues including intestine under hypoxic conditions (9). However, HIF-2α has not been investigated in intestinal ischaemia.

In the horse, intestinal strangulation with concurrent ischaemia is a major cause of mortality (10). To the authors' knowledge, both HIF-1α and -2α expression or distribution have not been investigated in ischaemic intestinal tissue in the horse, yet the HIF-1α distribution has been investigated in small intestinal tissue oral or aboral to strangulating lesions (11). One author reported decreased HIF-1α expression in manipulated tissue compared to control samples (11), while another found no difference in HIF-1α expression (12)

Ischaemic postconditioning (IPoC) is the reocclusion of blood supply after abolishing a primary ischaemic insult. It has been shown to ameliorate ischaemia/reperfusion injury and represents a therapeutic strategy for ischaemic conditions in different tissues (13, 14). It has been suggested that HIF-1α plays a signalling role in the protective action of IPoC. In experimental models of intestinal and myocardial ischaemia in rodents, HIF-1α expression was higher in groups subjected to IPoC compared to the untreated control groups, and was associated with less tissue damage (14-16). In contrast, one study investigating IPoC in myocardial ischaemia showed that the protective function of ischaemic post-conditioning was mediated by down-regulation of HIF-1α (17).

The aim of this study was to investigate the distribution of hypoxia inducible factors 1α and -2α in experimental small intestinal ischaemia in horses. A second objective was to evaluate the role of hypoxia inducible factors in ischaemic postconditioning in an equine model of segmental jejunal ischaemia. The authors hypothesized that HIF-1α and HIF-2α levels would increase during ischaemia and reperfusion, and that this would be more pronounced in the animals subjected to postconditioning.

Materials and Methods

Experimental design

The study was reviewed by the Ethics Committee for Animal Experiments of Lower Saxony, Germany, and approved according to §8 of the German Animal Welfare Act (LAVES 33.8-42502-04-18/2856). A power analysis was performed prior to commencing the study using free available software (G*Power 3.1.9.2, *Heinrich Heine Universität, Düsseldorf, Germany*). To detect a difference in immunohistochemistry score with an effect size of 1.5, a sample size of 7 horses per treatment group was required, based on a power of 0.8 and alpha of 0.05. Fourteen horses, owned by the university, were randomly assigned to a group subjected to postconditioning (group IPoC; n=7) and an untreated control group (group C, n=7).

Animals

All horses were systemically healthy, and had been elected for euthanasia due to severe orthopaedic problems. The horses were stabled at the facilities of the university at least two weeks prior to surgery. The horses had free access to hay and water and were hand walked daily. Group C consisted of five Warmbloods, one Islandic horse and one Thoroughbred, with a mean age of 12.6 ± 8.7 years and mean weight of 535 ± 89 kg. Group IPoC consisted of four Warmbloods, one Islandic pony, one Thoroughbred, and one Standardbred, with a mean age of 10.4 ± 8.6 years and weight of 506 ± 96 kg.

Anaesthesia and surgical procedure

General anaesthesia was induced with 0.1 mg/kg BW diazepam (Ziapam 5 mg/kg, *Ecuphar GmbH, Greifswald, Germany*) and 2.2 mg/kg ketamine (Narketan, *Vétoquinol GmbH, Ismaning, Germany*) after premedication with 0.7 mg/kg body weight (BW) xylazine (Xylavet 20 mg/ml, *CP-Pharma GmbH, Burgdorf, Germany*). Anaesthesia was maintained with isoflurane (Isofluran CP, *CP-Pharma GmbH*) in 100% oxygen, and continuous rate infusions with lactated Ringer's solution (Ringer-Laktat EcobagClick, *B. Braun Melsungen AG, Melsungen, Germany*) and dobutamine (Dobutamin-ratiopharm 250mg, *Ratiopharm GmbH, Ulm, Germany*) were given to effect, to maintain the mean arterial blood pressure between 60 and 80 mmHg. A routine pre-umbilical median laparotomy was performed in dorsal recumbency. Segmental small intestinal ischaemia was induced in 1.5 m jejunum by occlusion of the mesenteric vessels with umbilical tape. The ligature was tightened under monitoring of the intestinal microperfusion with microlightguide spectophotometry and laser Doppler flowmetry (O_2C, *LEA Medizintechnik GmbH, Giessen, Germany*), and the ligature was tied when the blood flow was reduced by 90% of the preischaemic measurement. The ischaemia was maintained for 90 min. In group C, the ligature was released without manipulation of the vessels or the intestine. In group IPoC, postconditioning was implemented after release of ischaemia by clamping the mesenteric vessels for 3 cycles of 30 sec, alternated with 30 sec of reperfusion. This was followed by 120 minutes of reperfusion in both groups. Subsequently, the horses were euthanized without regaining consciousness.

Sample collection and preparation

Full thickness intestinal samples were taken at the end of the pre-ischaemia period (pre-ischaemia sample, P), at the end of ischaemia (ischaemia sample, I), and at the end of reperfusion (reperfusion sample, R). At this time point, an additional sample was taken just proximal to the post-ischaemic intestinal segment (proximal sample, PR). One segment of each sample was fixed in a 4% formaldehyde solution for 24 to 36 hours and subsequently embedded in paraffin.

Immunohistochemical staining was performed for HIF1α and HIF2α. In short, the slides were deparaffinized and subsequently the antigens were demasked in a citrate buffer with a pH of 6.0 at 95 °C for 20 min, followed by blocking for unspecific binding with 20 % goat serum. The slides were incubated overnight with 1:500 polyclonal rabbit antibody against HIF1α (HIF-1 alpha Antibody NB100-134, Novus Biologicals LLC, Centennial USA) or 1:100 monoclonal mouse anti-body against HIF2α (Anti-Hypoxia Inducible Factor 2 α Antibody clone 190b, *Sigma Aldrich, Darmstadt, Germany).* Subsequently, the slides were incubated with secondary antibody (1:200 goat-anti-rabbit or 1:200 goat-anti-mouse, respectively), followed by incubation with the ABC reagent (Vectastain ABC, *Biozol diagnostics Vertrieb GmbH, Eching, Germany*). The negative control was incubated with 1:3000 rabbit serum (R4505, *Sigma Aldrich Merck KGaA, Darmstadt, Germany*) in PBS with 1% BSA instead of the primary antibody for HIF1α, and with 1:30 Mouse IgG1 for HIF2α. Equine kidney tissue and equine squamous cell carcinoma tissue was used as a positive control. The slides were incubated with 3,3′-diaminobenzidine and counterstained with modified hematoxylin (Delafield Hemalaun).

All slides were scanned to a digital format at 20x magnification (Axio Scan.Z1, *Carl Zeiss GmbH, Oberkochen, Germany*), and subsequently evaluated using the accompanying software (Zen Blue 3.0, *Carl Zeiss GmbH*). In addition to the descriptive evaluation, a semi-quantitative score was developed for comparison between the groups and time-points. The enterocytes in the crypts and the villus were graded separately for staining intensity of both the cytoplasm and the nucleus with the following score for immunoreactivity: 0 – no staining; 1 – weak staining (very light brown); 2 – mild staining (light brown); 3 – moderate staining (medium brown); 4 – intense staining (dark brown). To quantify the difference between the cytoplasmic and nuclear staining within one slide, the nucleus/cytoplasm ratio was calculated. The same score was used for the myocytes of the tunica muscularis. Microscopic photographs were used as colour reference, and the evaluation was performed at fixed colour settings by one observer, who was blinded for the identity of the slides. Because of the observation that many sections showed a varying amount of focal cytoplasmic staining close to the nucleus, a separate score was implemented to quantify the proportion of cells with this perinuclear staining: 0 – < 1%; 1 – 1% to 25%; 2 – 26% to 50%; 3 – 51% to 75%; 4 – 76% to 100%.

Data Analysis

Statistical analysis and graph design were performed using commercial software (Graphpad Prism 8.4.2, *Graphpad Software Inc., San Diego, California, USA*). The results of the semi-quantitative score were expressed as median (min-max). For comparison of this score between the groups and time-points, distribution free nonparametric models were used for independent (treatment and control group) and correlated (time points) effects. A Mann-Whitney-U test was executed to compare the results between the different groups at each time point. For comparing the correlated different time points, a Friedman test in combination with the post hoc Dunns-test for multiple pairwise comparisons was performed. Alpha was set at 0.05.

Results

HIF-1α immunohistochemistry

The enterocytes exhibited a mild to moderate cytoplasmic and a mild to intense nuclear staining (Fig. 1A and B). Inflammatory cells, endothelial cells, and interstitial cells showed consistent intense nuclear staining. In most slides, the crypt enterocytes showed more nuclear and cytoplasmic staining than the villus enterocytes. In some of the pre-ischaemia and PR samples with long villi, a more intense staining at the tip of the villus was observed compared to the middle and base section. A varying proportion of crypt enterocytes exhibited a perinucleur focal accumulation of intense staining (Fig. 1C). In the villus enterocytes, a similar phenomenon was observed in some of the samples, with moderate to intense focal perinuclear staining, predominantly seen at the base of the villus (Fig. 1D). However, the majority showed only diffuse staining of the cytoplasm. The neurons of the submucosa and myenteric plexi showed moderate to intense nuclear staining (Fig. 1E). In the tunica muscularis, the myocytes showed moderate to intense nuclear and mild to moderate cytoplasmic staining (Fig. 1F), sometimes with a patchy appearance.

There were no significant differences between the HIF-1α staining scores of the two groups. Therefore, the samples of both groups were pooled for comparison between the different time points (Table 1). The reperfusion samples had a significantly higher score for cytoplasmic staining of both the crypts (median difference 1, p = 0.047) and the villi (median difference 0.5, p = 0.016) compared to pre-ischaemia. The nuclear staining in the villus enterocytes was also higher in the reperfusion sample (median difference 1, p = 0.0081). The score for perinuclear granules in the crypt enterocyte cytoplasm was significantly lower after reperfusion compared to pre-ischaemia (median difference 1, p = 0.0038), as was the nucleus/cytoplasm ratio in the crypts (median difference 0.5, p = 0.031).

Table 1. HIF-1α immunoreactivity score in the equine jejunum during experimental I/R injury

	Crypt				***Villus***				***Muscularis***	
Control group	*Cytoplasm*	*Nucleus*	*Nucl./cytopl.*	*Perinuclear*	*Cytoplasm*	*Nucleus*	*Nucl./cytopl.*	*Perinuclear*	*Cytoplasm*	*Nucleus*
Pre-ischaemia	2 (2 - 3)	4 (3 - 4)	1.5 (1.3 - 2)	2 (0 - 2)	2 (1 - 2)	2 (1 - 2)	1 (0.5 - 2)	0 (0 - 3)	3 (2 - 3)	4 (4)
Ischaemia	3 (2 - 4)	4 (3 - 4)	1.3 (1 - 2)	1 (0 - 3)	2 (2 - 3)	3 (1 - 3)	1 (0.5 - 1.5)	0 (0 - 3)	3 (2 - 3)	4 (4)
Reperfusion	3 (2 - 4)	4 (4)	1.3 (1 - 2)	0 (0 - 1)	3 (2 - 4)	3 (2 - 4)	1 (0.7 - 1.5)	0 (0 - 2)	2 (2 - 3)	4 (4)
Proximal	2 (2 - 3)	4 (3 - 4)	1.3 (1.3-1.5)	1 (0 - 1)	2 (2)	2 (1 - 3)	1 (0.5 - 1.5)	0 (0 - 3)	3 (0 - 3)	4 (0 - 4)

	Crypt				***Villus***				***Muscularis***	
IPoC group	*Cytoplasm*	*Nucleus*	*Nucl./cytopl.*	*Perinuclear*	*Cytoplasm*	*Nucleus*	*Nucl./cytopl.*	*Perinuclear*	*Cytoplasm*	*Nucleus*
Pre-ischaemia	2 (2 - 3)	4 (4)	2 (1.3 - 2)	2 (1 - 3)	2 (2)	2 (2 - 3)	1 (1 - 1.5)	1 (0 - 2)	3 (3)	4 (4)
Ischaemia	3 (2 - 4)	4 (3 - 4)	1.3 (1 - 1.5)	1 (0 - 3)	2 (1 - 2)	2 (2 - 3)	1 (1 - 2)	1 (0 - 3)	2 (2 - 3)	4 (3 - 4)
Reperfusion	3 (2 - 4)	4 (4)	1.3 (1 - 2)	1 (0 - 2)	2 (2 - 3)	3 (2 - 4)	1.5 (1 - 2)	0 (0 - 2)	2 (2 - 3)	4 (3 - 4)
Proximal	2 (2 - 4)	4 (4)	2 (1 - 2)	1 (0 - 3)	2 (2 - 3)	3 (1 - 3)	1 (0.5 - 1.5)	1 (0 - 3)	2 (2 - 3)	4 (4)

	Crypt				***Villus***				***Muscularis***	
Total	*Cytoplasm*	*Nucleus*	*Nucl./cytopl.*	*Perinuclear*	*Cytoplasm*	*Nucleus*	*Nucl./cytopl.*	*Perinuclear*	*Cytoplasm*	*Nucleus*
Pre-ischaemia	2 (2 - 3)	4 (3 - 4)	1.8 (1.3 - 2)	2 (0 - 3)	2 (1 - 2)	2 (1 - 3)	1 (0.5 - 2)	0 (0 - 3)	3 (3)	4 (4)
Ischaemia	3 (2 - 4)	4 (3 - 4)	1.3 (1 - 2)	1 (0 - 3)	2 (1 - 3)	2 (1 - 3)	1 (0.5 - 2)	1 (0 - 3)	3 (2 - 3)	4 (3 - 4)
Reperfusion	3 (2 - 4)*	4 (4)	1.3 (1 - 2)*	1 (0 - 2)*	2.5(2 - 4)*	3 (2-4)**	1.2 (0.7 - 2)	0 (0 - 2)	2 (2 - 3)	4 (3 - 4)
Proximal	2 (2 - 4)	4 (3 - 4)	1.5 (1 - 2)	1 (0 - 3)	2 (2 - 3)	2 (1 - 3)	1 (0.5 - 1.5)	1 (0 - 3)	3 (2 - 3)	4 (0 - 4)

The table displays the median (minimum – maximum) score. The asterisks indicate a significant difference compared to the pre-ischaemia sample of that variable (= p<0.05; ** = p<0.01).*

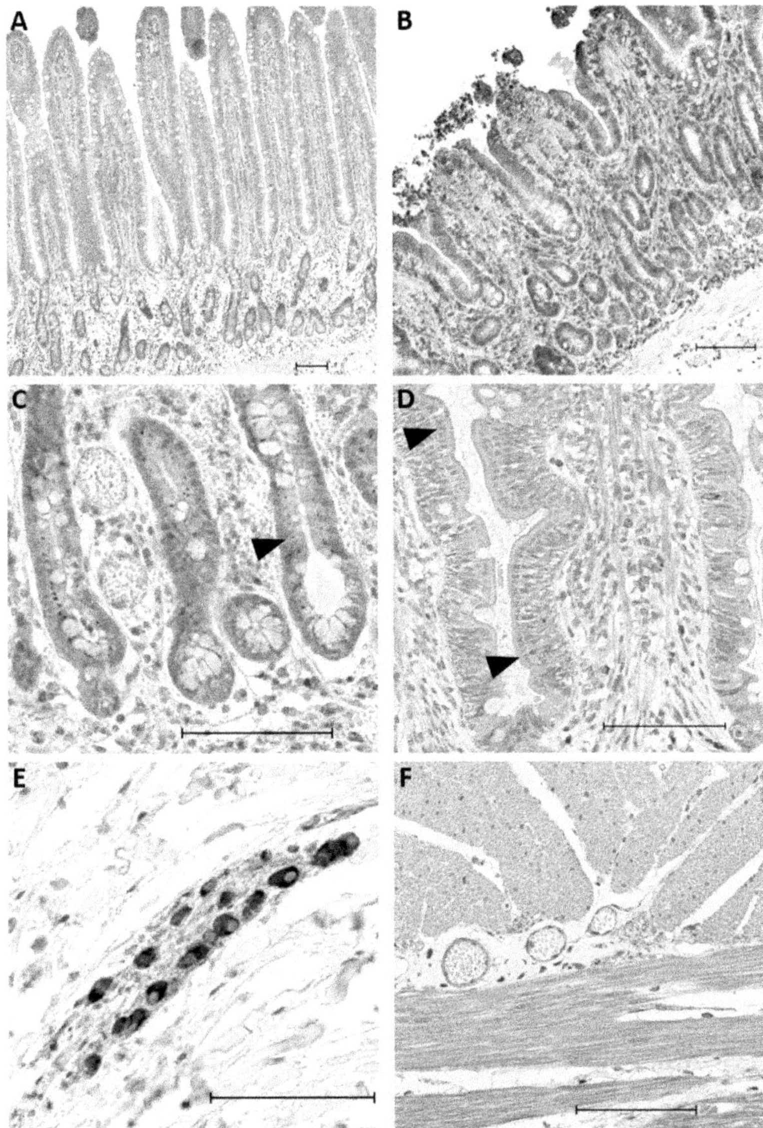

Figure 1: Microscopic images of HIF-1α stained sections showing representative examples of the immunoreactivity patterns in the jejunum of horses subjected to experimental ischaemia. (A) Intestinal mucosa of a pre-ischaemia sample, demonstrating more intense enterocyte staining in the crypts compared to the villus; (B) intestinal mucosa belonging to the same horse as sample A, taken after reperfusion; (C) crypt enterocytes with intense focal perinuclear staining (arrowheads); (D) villus enterocytes with moderate perinuclear focal staining in a preíschaemia sample (arrowheads); (E) neurons of the submucosa plexus with intense staining; (F) myocytes in the tunica muscularis with moderate - intense nuclear staining and moderate myoplasmic staining. The scale bar indicates 100 µm.

HIF-2α immunohistochemistry

In general, there was less intense staining of the sections after *HIF-2α IHC* compared to HIF-1α. The enterocytes showed no nuclear and weak to moderate cytoplasmic staining. In the villus, comparable to the HIF-1α stained sections, the enterocytes exhibited 2 different staining patterns. Most commonly, a diffuse staining of the cytoplasm was seen (Fig. 2A and B). In some of the sections, all the villus enterocytes exhibited a moderate – intense focal staining just apical to the nucleus (Fig. 2C and D). Subjectively, this appeared to be more intense and crescent shapes at the erosion fronts of some of the villi in the ischaemia and reperfusion samples. However, this was not a consistent finding. In the crypts, there where varying amounts of cells with intense perinuclear staining in the enterocytes and goblet cells (Fig. 2E). In some of the cells, this focal intense staining formed a crescent shape around the nucleus. The endothelial cells, leucocytes and stromal cells demonstrated weak staining in the majority of the slides. The neurons in the submucosal and myenteric plexi were weak to moderately stained (Fig. 2F). The myocytes in the tunica muscularis showed a weak to mild cytoplasmic and nuclear staining (Fig. 2F). Furthermore, varying amounts of moderate to intense stained granules could be observed, mostly located perinuclear (Fig. 2F). In the serosa of the reperfusion and proximal samples, some of the neutrophils demonstrated a moderate staining cytoplasmic and nuclear staining.

The HIF-2α immunoreactivity scores can be seen in Table 2, excluding the nuclear score, as these were all zero for this stain. There were no significant differences between the groups or time points.

Table 2 HIF-2α immunoreactivity score in the equine jejunum during experimental I/R injury

	Crypt		***Villus***		***Muscularis***	
Control group	*Cytoplasm*	*Perinuclear*	*Cytoplasm*	*Perinuclear*	*Cytoplasm*	*Perinuclear*
Pre-ischaemia	1 (0 - 3)	2 (1 - 3)	2 (0 - 3)	1 (0 - 4)	3 (1 - 3)	2 (1 - 3)
Ischaemia	1 (1 - 2)	3 (1 - 4)	2 (1 - 3)	1 (0 - 4)	1 (1 - 3)	2 (0 - 2)
Reperfusion	1 (1 - 2)	2 (1 - 4)	2 (1 - 3)	1 (0 - 4)	2 (1 - 2)	1 (1 - 3)
proximal	1 (1 - 2)	2 (1 - 4)	2 (1 - 3)	0 (0 - 4)	1 (0 - 3)	1 (0 - 3)
	Crypt		***Villus***		***Muscularis***	
IPoC group	*Cytoplasm*	*Perinuclear*	*Cytoplasm*	*Perinuclear*	*Cytoplasm*	*Perinuclear*
Pre-ischaemia	1 (1 - 2)	2 (1 - 4)	2 (1 - 3)	1 (0 - 4)	2 (1 - 2)	2 (0 - 3)
Ischaemia	1 (1 - 2)	2 (1 - 4)	2 (1 - 3)	1 (0 - 4)	1 (1 - 2)	1 (1 - 3)
Reperfusion	1 (1 - 2)	2 (1 - 4)	2 (1 - 2)	1 (0 - 4)	1 (1 - 2)	1 (0 - 2)
proximal	1 (1 - 2)	2 (1 - 4)	2 (1 - 3)	1 (0 - 4)	1 (1 - 2)	1 (0 - 2)
	Crypt		***Villus***		***Muscularis***	
Total	*Cytoplasm*	*Perinuclear*	*Cytoplasm*	*Perinuclear*	*Cytoplasm*	*Perinuclear*
Pre-ischaemia	1 (0 - 3)	2 (1 - 4)	2 (0 - 3)	1 (0 - 4)	2 (1 - 3)	2 (0 - 3)
Ischaemia	1 (1 - 2)	2.5 (1 - 4)	2 (1 - 3)	1 (0 - 4)	1 (1 - 3)	1.5 (0 - 3)
Reperfusion	1 (1 - 2)	2 (1 - 4)	2 (1 - 3)	1 (0 - 4)	1 (1 - 2)	1 (0 - 3)
Proximal	1 (1 - 2)	2 (1 - 4)	2 (1 - 3)	0.5 (0 - 4)	1 (0 - 3)	1 (0 - 3)

The table displays the median (minimum – maximum) score. There were no significant differences between the groups or time points.

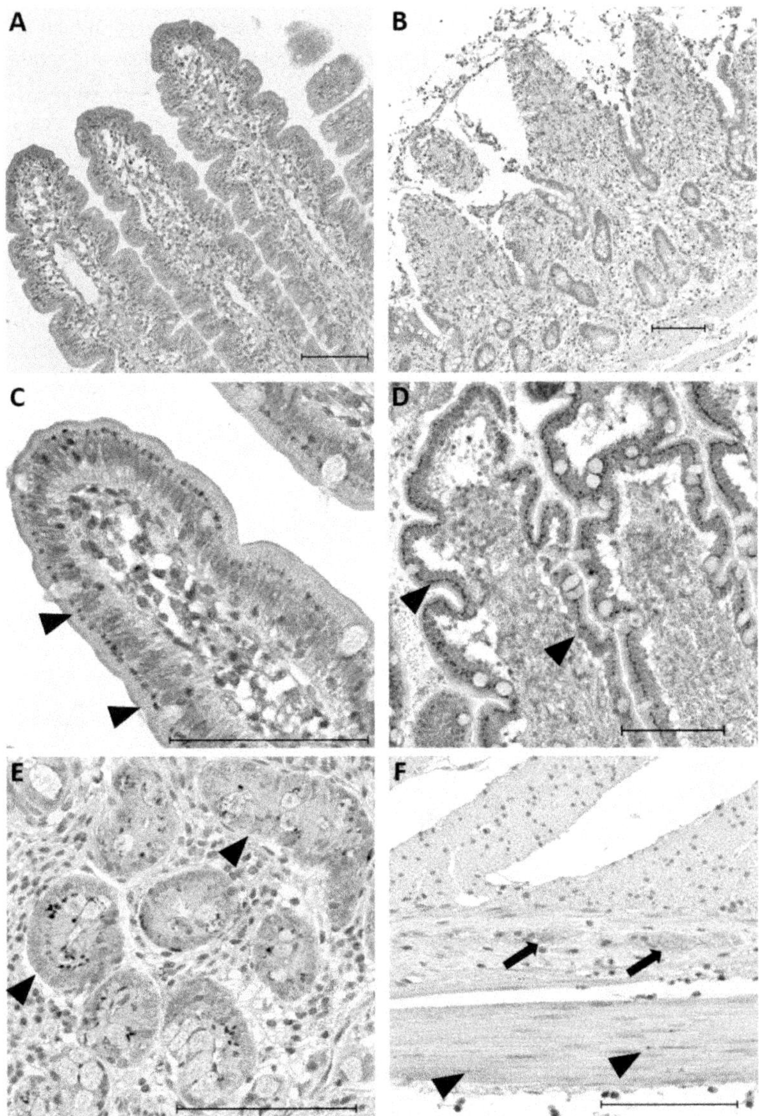

Figure 2: Microscopic images of HIF-2α stained sections showing representative examples of the immunoreactivity patterns in the jejunum of horses subjected to experimental ischaemia. The bar indicates 100 µm. (A) Mucosal villus enterocytes with diffuse mild cytoplasmic staining during pre-ischaemia; (B) Mucosa of the same horse after ischaemia, showing similar mild cytoplasmic staining in the remaining villus enterocytes; (C) Focal perinuclear intense staining in villus enterocytes during pre-ischaemia (arrowhead); (D) Mucosa of the same horse after ischaemia, showing similar intense perinuclear staining of the enterocytes (arrowhead); (E) Crypt enterocytes with diffuse weak cytoplasmic and focal perinuclear intense staining (arrowhead); (F) neurons in the myenteric plexus with mild staining (arrow) and myocytes in the tunica muscularis with weak diffuse staining and few intensely stained granules (arrowhead).

Remarkably, there were three horses (one from group C, two from group IPoC) which exhibited a focal intense cytoplasmic staining in all villus enterocytes (Fig. 2D and E), which was consistent throughout the samples of different time-points (Fig. 3A). On the contrary, the other 11 horses all exhibited scores of 0 or 1 (<25%) for perinuclear focal staining (Fig. 3A). Comparably, these three horses had median scores of 4 for the crypt perinuclear focal staining while the other horses had a median of 2 (Fig. 3B).

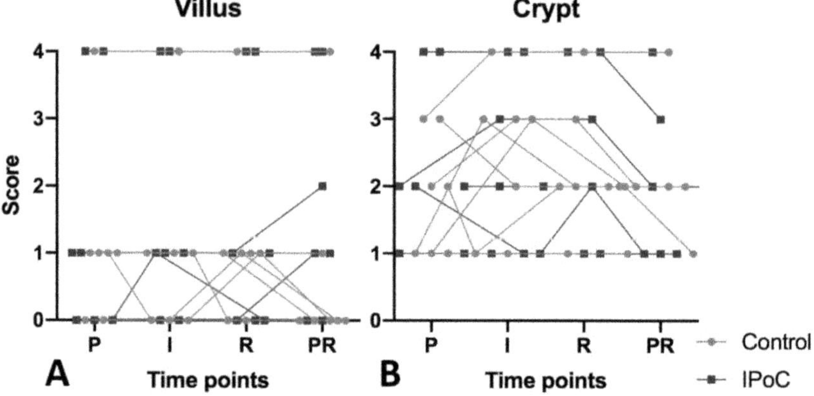

Figure 3: Connected individual value plots of the semi-quantitative score for focal perinuclear staining with Hypoxia Inducible 2-alpha in the small intestinal villus enterocytes (A) and crypt enterocytes (B) of 14 horses subjected to experimental jejunal ischaemia. IPoC is the group of horses undergoing ischaemia postconditioning, and the control group did not undergo any form of treatment. No differences between the groups could be detected. Three individual horses show consistent high scores for perinuclear staining, that do not change over time. P = Pre-ischaemia, I = Ischaemia, R = Reperfusion, PR = Proximal intestinal segment at reperfusion.

Discussion

This is the first study assessing the immunoreactivity pattern of hypoxia inducible factors HIF-1α and -2α in intestinal ischaemia in the horse. The main finding was that the intestinal mucosa showed an increased HIF-1α immunoreactivity score after reperfusion compared to pre-ischaemia. Contrarily, HIF-2α did not show any progression during ischaemia or reperfusion. Therefore, we could only partially accept our hypothesis that HIF-1α and HIF-2α levels would increase during ischaemia and reperfusion. We could not detect a difference in HIF-1α and -2α immunoreactivity between the treatment groups, rejecting the hypothesis that the HIF response would be more pronounced in the animal subjected to postconditioning.

Evaluating the HIF-1α distribution in the intestine, some degree of staining was present in all cell types, as previously reported in the equine small intestine (11). The increased immunoreactivity score over time correlates with a study in rats that increased numbers of positive cells are seen in injured villi (18). This study also reported many positive cells in the erosion fronts (18), which was not a predominant finding in the current study. We found the phenomenon of perinuclear focal HIF-1α immunoreactivity in a varying proportion of villus and crypt enterocytes. A granular pattern in the cytoplasm has previously been reported in the colon (19) and liver (20). This phenomenon may represent the accumulation of this protein in cytosolic vesicles. One study investigating HIF-1α in cell cultures, localized the transcription factor in the sub-membranous compartment and within cytosolic vesicles. This was linked to a reduced activation of its downstream pathway indicating a non-functional HIF-1α variant in response to decreased cytoplasmic degradation (21). This concept could apply to the enterocytes in the current study, although this cannot be concluded without further investigation.

The score for the perinuclear focal staining in the crypt enterocyte cytoplasm was significantly lower after reperfusion compared to pre-ischaemia. This could be associated with the increased diffuse cytoplasmic staining seen at this time-point, possibly indicating a shift from a focal collection or vesicle to cytoplasmic diffusion. Alternatively, this could be unrelated, and the increased cytoplasmic staining after reperfusion may be the result of HIF-1α upregulation. Increased nuclear staining with HIF-1α would be expected after ischaemia, because of transport from the cytosol to the nucleus as transcription factor (22). In the current study, an increased nuclear staining was found only in the villus. This may be explained by the higher level of hypoxia that is to be expected in the mucosal villus compared to the crypts (23). On the other hand, the crypt enterocytes had a higher staining intensity to begin with, limiting the possibility of a further increase.

Interestingly, the increased nuclear and cytoplasmic staining was not seen directly after ischaemia, but after 2 hours of reperfusion. Comparing this to the available literature, other studies have demonstrated increased intestinal protein expression 2 h to 12 h after hypoxia (6, 14, 24). Upregulation with increased mRNA levels has been shown to reach the maximum during the ischaemic phase (25). However, most research has been done in cell cultures under hypoxic conditions, instead of in vivo in an ischaemia model, complicating a direct comparison. Another explanation for the delayed HIF-1α increase, may lie in the significant association that has been described between HIF-1α expression and inflammatory infiltrates and cytokine release (26, 27). We found that the reperfusion samples exhibited the highest neutrophil counts during reperfusion, possibly eliciting a more pronounced HIF-1α response at this time point.

To quantify the difference between the cytoplasmic and nuclear staining within one slide, the nucleus/cytoplasm ratio was calculated. Here, the main finding was that this ratio was significantly lower in the crypts after reperfusion, reflecting the higher cytoplasmic staining combined with an absence in nuclear increased staining during this time point.

The proximal sample taken after reperfusion did not differ from the pre-ischaemia sample. Two studies that also investigated the HIF-1a response in intestine peripheral to an ischaemic lesion, reported differing results. One found that the manipulated tissues demonstrated significantly less HIF-1α expression in the tunica muscularis at 4 hours compared to the control tissues (11), and another found no difference between the peripheral segment and control samples (12). Therefore, the HIF-response in the proximal segment remains unclear.

The HIF-2α immunoreactivity pattern demonstrated mainly cytoplasmic staining of the enterocytes. The majority of the stromal cells were negative, similar to the results of a rodent study (9). This study also reported weak and inconsistent staining in the jejunum compared to the duodenum. This comparison could not be made in the current study, as only jejunum samples were taken. Interestingly, no significant change in immunoreactivity could be noted over time. The only finding that seemed related to the time point, was the incidental change in perinuclear staining in the villus enterocytes at epithelial erosion fronts. However, this was not consistently present, and it may also be related to the intracellular changes that occur at the time of epithelial separation, without a direct effect of HIF-2α itself. These results suggest that HIF-2α is not of significance in the hypoxia signaling in the current model of intestinal ischaemia in horses. On the other hand, this was determined by a semi-quantitative scale only. The duration of reperfusion may also be of significance, considering upregulation may require longer than the 2 hours of reperfusion implemented in the current study. One study in rats did report increased intestinal HIF-2α expression in response to CO within 1 h (9), thereby suggesting otherwise.

Another significant finding of current study was that no nuclear staining of HIF-2α was observed. Absence of nuclear staining with concurrent cytoplasmic HIF-2α staining has been reported in benign human ovarian tumors (28). Therefore, this is not an unlikely finding, and possibly suggests a lack of activity of this transcription factor in the applied animal model. However, there are no comparable intestinal histological studies or studies in in vivo ischaemia models, limiting further comparison of results.

Three of 14 horses exhibited a consistent and distinct intense perinuclear staining pattern in nearly all enterocytes throughout all samples, whereas other horses demonstrated perinuclear staining in only a small proportion of the enterocytes. Nearly all samples also demonstrated a granular HIF-2α immunoreactivity in the tunica muscularis. As discussed for the HIF-1α results, this staining pattern may represent the assembly in vesicles. The fact that all samples of these individuals showed the same distribution, independent of timing or ischaemia, suggests an association with the individual horses and not with the experimental model. It has been shown that HIF-2α expression can be related to age, with lower levels in aged gingival tissues (29). However, looking at age, breed and sex of these three horses, no explanation could be found for the different HIF-2α distribution pattern. The horses did not differ from the other animals in degree of mucosal injury or inflammation. Furthermore, there were no disparities in test group, timing of the experiment, involved personnel or sample processing. Therefore, the cause this for phenomenon remains unresolved, and requires further investigation.

A direct comparison between the HIF-1α and -2α scores was not performed, because the difference in antibody type (monoclonal vs. polyclonal) and dilution would preclude a reliable comparison. Nevertheless, looking at the immunoreactivity patterns of both factors, clear differences could be identified. Firstly, nuclear immunoreactivity for HIF-1α was seen in all cell types, while there was no nuclear staining for HIF-2α. Furthermore, HIF-1α showed more intense staining in the crypts compared to the villi, yet for HIF-2α this was the other way around. Moreover, the HIF-2α stained slides exhibited a higher proportion of enterocytes with focal perinuclear staining, and the focal granular staining in the tunica muscularis was only found in these slides.

Previous studies have found evidence for upregulation of HIF-1α being of significance for the protective action of IPC and IPoC in laboratory animals (14, 16, 30). It was reported that HIF-1α was higher after both intestinal and cardiac IPoC, with subsequent upregulation of microRNA-21 as mediator (14, 16). Contrarily, another study investigating IPoC in myocardial ischaemia showed that microRNA-214 may participate in the protective function of IPoC by down-regulating HIF-1α (17). These conflicting results indicate that the association between HIF-1α and the protective action of ischaemic conditioning is not set in stone. In the current study, we could not find a significant difference between the control group and the group undergoing postconditioning. In our previous study with the same samples, we found some indicators for a protective effect of IPoC, yet the parameters for oxidative stress did not differ between the groups. This could possibly account for the absence of an effect on HIF-1α, considering the relationship between the HIF-1α response and oxidative stress (22, 31).

The main limitation of this study is the semi-quantitative nature of the results, possibly limiting the detection of smaller differences. A quantitative protein analysis and RNA analysis would give more information on this matter, is currently in progress. Immunohistology scores may be prone to subjectivity and there was only one observer. Nevertheless, the slides were reviewed in a blinded manner, and an observer bias would be present in all samples. Furthermore, reference microscopic images were used to standardize this evaluation.

In conclusion, the mucosal changes in HIF-1α immunoreactivity over time indicate that this transcription factor plays a role in the intestinal response to ischaemia. HIF-2α did not show any progression during ischaemia or reperfusion and no nuclear staining was observed, suggesting that this transcription factor does not modulate the effect of hypoxia in small intestinal ischaemia. A distinct perinuclear focal HIF-2α staining pattern was associated with individual horses and not with time points, requiring further investigation. We could not detect a difference in HIF-1α and -2α immunoreactivity between the treatment groups, possibly indicating that these factors are not relevant for postconditioning in the current experimental model. More research including quantitative analysis and downstream target levels is needed to assess the exact role of HIF expression in the equine intestine.

References

(1) Tirpe AA, Gulei D, Ciortea SM, Crivii C, Berindan-Neagoe I. Hypoxia: overview on hypoxia-mediated mechanisms with a focus on the role of HIF genes. International Journal of Molecular Sciences. 2019;20(24):6140.

(2) Semenza GL. Regulation of mammalian O2 homeostasis by hypoxia-inducible factor 1. Annual review of cell and developmental biology. 1999;15(1):551-78.

(3) Grenz A, Clambey E, Eltzschig HK. Hypoxia signaling during intestinal ischemia and inflammation. Curr Opin Crit Care. 2012;18(2):178-85.

(4) Saeedi BJ, Kao DJ, Kitzenberg DA, Dobrinskikh E, Schwisow KD, Masterson JC, et al. HIF-dependent regulation of claudin-1 is central to intestinal epithelial tight junction integrity. Molecular biology of the cell. 2015;26(12):2252-62.

(5) Kannan KB, Colorado I, Reino D, Palange D, Lu Q, Qin X, et al. Hypoxia-inducible factor plays a gut-injurious role in intestinal ischemia reperfusion injury. American Journal of Physiology-Gastrointestinal and Liver Physiology. 2011;300(5):G853-G61.

(6) Feinman R, Deitch EA, Watkins AC, Abungu B, Colorado I, Kannan KB, et al. HIF-1 mediates pathogenic inflammatory responses to intestinal ischemia-reperfusion injury. American Journal of Physiology-Gastrointestinal and Liver Physiology. 2010;299(4):G833-G43.

(7) Knudsen AR, Kannerup A-S, Grønbæk H, Andersen KJ, Funch-Jensen P, Frystyk J, et al. Effects of ischemic pre-and postconditioning on HIF-1α, VEGF and TGF-β expression after warm ischemia and reperfusion in the rat liver. Comparative hepatology. 2011;10(1):3.

(8) Wang P, Qi H, Sun C, He W, Chen G, Li L, et al. Overexpression of hypoxia-inducible factor-1alpha exacerbates endothelial barrier dysfunction induced by hypoxia. Cell Physiol Biochem. 2013;32(4):859-70.

(9) Wiesener MS, Jürgensen JS, Rosenberger C, Scholze C, Hörstrup JH, Warnecke C, et al. Widespread, hypoxia-inducible expression of HIF-2α in distinct cell populations of different organs. The FASEB Journal. 2003;17(2):271-3.

(10) Tinker MK, White N, Lessard P, Thatcher C, Pelzer K, Davis B, et al. Prospective study of equine colic incidence and mortality. Equine veterinary journal. 1997;29(6):448-53.

(11) Bauck A. G.; Grosche A.: Morton AJG, A. S.; Vickroy, T. W.; Freeman, D. E. Effect of lidocaine on in ammation in equine jejunum subjected to manipulation only and remote to intestinal segments subjected to ischemia. AJVR. 2017;78(8):977 - 89.

(12) De Ceulaer K, Delesalle C, Van Elzen R, Van Brantegem L, Weyns A, Van Ginneken C. Morphological data indicate a stress response at the oral border of strangulated small intestine in horses. Res Vet Sci. 2011;91(2):294-300.

(13) Zhi-Qing Zhao JSC, Michael E. Halkos, Faraz Kerendi,, Ning-Ping Wang RAG, and Jakob Vinten-Johansen. Inhibition of myocardial injury by ischemic postconditioning duringreperfusion: comparison with ischemic preconditioning. Am J Physiol Heart Circ Physiol. 2003;285:579-88.

(14) Jia Z, Lian W, Shi H, Cao C, Han S, Wang K, et al. Ischemic Postconditioning Protects Against Intestinal Ischemia/Reperfusion Injury via the HIF-1alpha/miR-21 Axis. Sci Rep. 2017;7(1):16190.

(15) Zhao H-X, Wang X-L, Wang Y-H, Wu Y, Li X-Y, Lv X-P, et al. Attenuation of myocardial injury by postconditioning: role of hypoxia inducible factor-1α. Basic research in cardiology. 2010;105(1):109.

(16) Liu Y, Nie H, Zhang K, Ma D, Yang G, Zheng Z, et al. A feedback regulatory loop between HIF-1α and miR-21 in response to hypoxia in cardiomyocytes. FEBS letters. 2014;588(17):3137-46.

(17) Wan D, Zhang Z, Yang H. Cardioprotective effect of miR-214 in myocardial ischemic postconditioning by down-regulation of hypoxia inducible factor 1, alpha subunit inhibitor. Cellular and molecular biology (Noisy-le-Grand, France). 2015;61(2):1.

(18) Tuboly E, Futakuchi M, Varga G, Érces D, Tőkés T, Mészáros A, et al. C5a inhibitor protects against ischemia/reperfusion injury in rat small intestine. Microbiology and immunology. 2016;60(1):35-46.

(19) Mariani F, Sena P, Marzona L, Riccio M, Fano R, Manni P, et al. Cyclooxygenase-2 and hypoxia-inducible factor-1α protein expression is related to inflammation, and up-regulated since the early steps of colorectal carcinogenesis. Cancer letters. 2009;279(2):221-9.

(20) Li S, Yao D, Wang L, Wu W, Qiu L, Yao M, et al. Expression characteristics of hypoxia-inducible factor-1α and its clinical values in diagnosis and prognosis of hepatocellular carcinoma. Hepatitis monthly. 2011;11(10):821-8.

(21) Armando F, Gambini M, Corradi A, Giudice C, Pfankuche VM, Brogden G, et al. Oxidative Stress in Canine Histiocytic Sarcoma Cells Induced by an Infection with Canine Distemper Virus Led to a Dysregulation of HIF-1α Downstream Pathway Resulting in a Reduced Expression of VEGF-B In Vitro. Viruses. 2020;12(2):200.

(22) Krock BL, Skuli N, Simon MC. Hypoxia-induced angiogenesis: good and evil. Genes & cancer. 2011;2(12):1117-33.

(23) Blikslager AT. The Equine Acute Abdomen: John Wiley & Sons; 2017.

(24) Ji Z-P, Li Y-X, Shi B-X, Zhuang Z-N, Yang J-Y, Guo S, et al. Hypoxia preconditioning protects Ca2+-ATPase activation of intestinal mucosal cells against R/I injury in a rat liver transplantation model. World Journal of Gastroenterology. 2018;24(3):360.

(25) Nishie H, Takahashi T, Inoue K, Shimizu H, Morimatsu H, Toda Y, et al. Site-specific induction of intestinal hypoxia-inducible factor-1α after hemorrhagic shock. Molecular medicine reports. 2009;2(2):149-52.

(26) Scharte M, Han X, Bertges DJ, Fink MP, Delude RL. Cytokines induce HIF-1 DNA binding and the expression of HIF-1-dependent genes in cultured rat enterocytes. American Journal of Physiology-Gastrointestinal and Liver Physiology. 2003;284(3):G373-G84.

(27) Garcia-Vasquez C, Fernandez-Acenero MJ, Garcia Gomez-Heras S, Pastor C. Fibrin patch influences the expression of hypoxia-inducible factor-1alpha and nuclear factor-kappaBp65 factors on ischemic intestinal anastomosis. Exp Biol Med (Maywood). 2018;243(10):803-8.

(28) Osada R, Horiuchi A, Kikuchi N, Yoshida J, Hayashi A, Ota M, et al. Expression of hypoxia-inducible factor 1α, hypoxia-inducible factor 2α, and von Hippel–Lindau protein in epithelial ovarian neoplasms and allelic loss of von Hippel-Lindau gene: nuclear expression of hypoxia-inducible factor 1α is an independent prognostic factor in ovarian carcinoma. Human pathology. 2007;38(9):1310-20.

(29) Ebersole JL, Novak MJ, Orraca L, Martinez-Gonzalez J, Kirakodu S, Chen KC, et al. Hypoxia-inducible transcription factors, HIF1A and HIF2A, increase in aging mucosal tissues. Immunology. 2018;154(3):452-64.

(30) Chen Y, Lee S-H, Tsai Y-H, Tseng S-H. Ischemic preconditioning increased the intestinal stem cell activities in the intestinal crypts in mice. Journal of Surgical Research. 2014;187(1):85-93.

(31) Movafagh S, Crook S, Vo K. Regulation of hypoxia-inducible factor-1a by reactive oxygen species: new developments in an old debate. Journal of cellular biochemistry. 2015;116(5):696-703.

9. Discussion

9.1. Main findings

The investigation into the preconditioning effect of lidocaine and xylazine did not reveal significant differences in the histomorphological changes between the treatment groups. Nonetheless, xylazine treatment resulted in the presence of fewer apoptotic and inflammatory cells in the mucosa and serosa after reperfusion compared to the control group. The group receiving lidocaine did not show any differences compared to the other groups, indicating that this treatment had no effect. Consequently, the results only partially support our first hypothesis that pharmacological preconditioning with lidocaine and xylazine ameliorates I/R injury.

In the evaluation of the implementation of IPoC, postconditioning clamping of the mesenteric vessels effectively reduced the intestinal microperfusion during all clamping cycles, yet affected tissue oxygen saturation only during the first cycle. The mesentery and its vessels did not show increased tissue damage after IPoC compared to the mesentery of the control group. The results support the hypothesis that IPoC is feasible and safe to perform; however, the chosen algorithm of clamping 3 cycles of 30 seconds did not effectively reduce the tissue oxygen saturation during later cycles.

Postconditioning resulted in reduced epithelial denudation and decreased paracellular permeability after reperfusion. However, IPoC did not affect electrophysiological variables and transcellular nutritional transport. Consequently, the results only partially support the hypothesis that intestinal mucosal morphology and function would be better preserved after IPoC.

The assessment of different markers for cell death, inflammation and oxidative stress showed that all evaluated parameters, apart from the neuronal cell counts in the myenteric plexus and the plasma levels of CK and LDH, changed significantly during ischaemia and/or reperfusion. Looking at the differences between the treatment groups, IPoC resulted in a lower apoptotic cell count after reperfusion, yet none of the other tested variables were significantly modified by this treatment. Accordingly, the results only partially support the hypothesis that IPoC decreases intestinal cell death, inflammation, and oxidative stress.

The intestinal expression and distribution of HSP-70 and hypoxia inducible factors -1α and -2α did not differ between the groups. This result does not support the initial hypothesis that IPoC is associated with a more pronounced heat shock and HIF response. Nevertheless, we observed an effect of the experimental model on the HSP-70 and HIF-1α immunoreactivity patterns of the enterocytes. Prior to ischaemia, HSP-70 was predominantly located in the cytoplasm, whereas after reperfusion, pronounced nuclear immunoreactivity was seen, suggesting translocation. The HIF-1α immunoreactivity scores were also significantly higher after reperfusion. In HIF-2α stained sections, however, no significant change in immunoreactivity was noted over time. A remarkable finding was that 3/14 horses exhibited a distinct intense perinuclear HIF-2α immunoreactivity of nearly all enterocytes in all samples and at all time points, while in the remaining horses this perinuclear staining was only observed in a small proportion of the enterocytes.

9.2. Interpretation of the results

9.2.1. The ischaemia model

The experimental model was effective in creating significant ischaemic injury within 90 minutes of 90% occlusion, as shown by the mucosal histomorphological changes in both experimental trials. The experimental model elicited consistent ischaemia between the groups, shown by similar intestinal microperfusion and oxygen saturation levels. Most tested variables showed some variability between individual horses, possibly due to biological variation or disparities in local blood flow. The venous and arterial blood flow in clinical strangulating obstructions may depend on the type and duration of the strangulation, and larger clinical studies investigating intestinal blood flow are lacking. Therefore, it remains difficult to establish a reliable and representative experimental model for equine strangulating colic.

Experimental studies investigating conditioning in rats, mice and pigs have reported an array of positive effects, and nearly all investigated variables were shown to benefit from conditioning therapy. Comparable to clinical trials in human patients (118), the present study has found certain beneficial effects, however, not to the same extent as in the experimental rodent models. This may be attributed to the difference in species, anaesthetic protocol, IPoC technique and ischaemia model.

Regarding the difference in species, there are several relevant differences between the intestine of horses and rodents. The levels of xanthine dehydrogenase - xanthine oxidase in the small intestine of horses are approximately 10-fold lower than those of rodents (25). Furthermore, horses have fewer resident mucosal neutrophils than rodents (197). This is relevant, as it has been suggested that the resident neutrophils in the mucosal lamina propria are responsible for most of the reperfusion injury (198). Therefore, rodents may be more prone to reperfusion injury. Contrarily, pigs appear to be more similar to horses, with comparable low levels of xanthine dehydrogenase - xanthine oxidase and resident neutrophils (199, 200). The effect of pre- and postconditioning would lie in the modulation of injury initiated during ischaemia, or the prevention of reperfusion injury (112). In regard to the latter, the significance of reperfusion injury in horses is under debate, based on several experimental studies and the above mentioned physiological factors (12, 197). This could limit the potential impact of IPoC and PPC in the horse. On the other hand, the increase in apoptotic and inflammatory cells during reperfusion in the current model suggests a significant effect of reperfusion. Furthermore, the studies investigating IPC and IPoC in pigs found significant protective effects in all tested variables (73, 141), indicating that low levels of xanthine dehydrogenase - xanthine oxidase and resident neutrophils may not be essential for effective conditioning. Species dependent variation in villus architecture and vessel anatomy could also be of significance (201).

Comparing the anaesthetic management, one realises that the rodents were predominantly anaesthetised with drugs that have not been investigated for a PPC effect such as ketamine and pentobarbital (79, 132, 138), whereas the horses in the current study all received isoflurane, known for its preconditioning effect. The latter may have elicited PPC protection in all groups, reducing the magnitude of the potential effect of the tested therapies. One study investigating cardiac IPC in rabbits confirmed that the anaesthetic protocol did affect the degree of infarct reduction by IPC (202). Animals anaesthetised with pentobarbital showed significantly more IPC dependent infarct reduction than those that received isoflurane or a combination of ketamine and xylazine. In contrast, it must be noted that there are several rodent studies investigating intestinal conditioning that have used ketamine and xylazine as anaesthetic agents, and still reported protective conditioning effects on all variables (130, 131, 134, 135). This suggests that an anaesthetic protocol with xylazine not necessarily interferes with the mechanism of conditioning in the rodent CMA occlusion model.

Regarding the different ischaemia models, it is evident that segmental jejunal ischaemia differs from the CMA occlusion model used in rodents. Blood flow studies in both rats and cats have shown that the CMA occlusion alone is associated with a highly variable degree of injury due to collateral circulation (203, 204). Furthermore, blood flow was shown to be reduced to a variable extent in the individual intestinal segments (203). Together with the fact that most reports did not mention from which intestinal area the samples were taken, this questions the reproducibility and reliability of the CMA model. The concept of segmental ischaemia may be more comparable to the small bowel transplantation models used in rats and pigs (92-95, 141). Nonetheless, the segmental jejunal ischaemia model used in the current experimental trial also comes with the risk of collateral circulation. However, this was managed adequately by the placement of additional oral and aboral ligatures. A possible advantage of segmental ischaemia could be that multiple ischaemic sections could be generated in one animal, as performed in one study on intestinal IPoC in rabbits (140). Yet with the knowledge that remote conditioning significantly affects peripheral injury (158), this strategy may be less suitable for studies investigating IPC and IPoC.

In summary, the multitude of differences between the experimental models renders a comparison between the studies difficult and emphasizes the importance of standardised experimental trials in the target species.

9.2.2. Feasibility of pre- and postconditioning in an experimental setting

In the present study, pharmacological preconditioning did not represent a challenge since the intravenous administration of drugs is routinely performed during anaesthetic management. To comply with the principle of hormesis, a preconditioning stimulus should mimic the effect of the following noxious event to elicit adaptive cellular responses. It is plausible that xylazine administration adheres to the concept of hormesis through the activation of adrenergic receptors with consecutive vasoconstriction and mimicking an ischaemic stimulus.

Lidocaine PPC may not adhere to this stricter definition of preconditioning. Its action is mediated by the blockade of voltage-dependent sodium channels (205) which is less likely to represent an ischaemic stimulus. We found no protective effect of lidocaine on any of the tested variables. Nevertheless, this does not exclude the use of this drug as therapeutic for I/R injury as we only tested a limited selection of parameters. Other studies in horses have reported multiple beneficial effects, such as analgesia (206), reduced intestinal oedema and mucosal permeability (53, 207), and decreased COX-2 expression in the intestinal mucosa (208). The only report in the literature of lidocaine in relation to pre- or postconditioning refers to its administration in combination with adenosine PPC for cardiac ischaemia in rats, resulting in an improved outcome, possibly through the abolishment of ventricular arrhythmias (209, 210). However, this mechanism of action would be less relevant for intestinal I/R injury.

For the implementation of IPoC, the use of modified haemostatic forceps proved to be a feasible technique in the equine jejunum, and the mesentery was not affected negatively by the clamping. The literature reports a broad range of re-occlusion times, with better results for the shorter durations of 5 – 10 seconds in rodents (130, 131, 134). For the current study, an algorithm of 3 cycles of 30 seconds was chosen, since a duration of 5 – 10 seconds was judged to be too short in this large species. We found that 30 seconds of clamping was sufficiently long to reduce the blood flow significantly, yet only the first clamping cycle led to significant tissue re-desaturation. This can most likely be explained by the short time span of flow reduction, combined with a swift recovery of oxygenation during the short bouts of reperfusion. We only measured the tissue oxygen saturation and not the oxygen pressure in the tissue. Undoubtedly, hypoxia would lead to desaturation; however, we do not know the exact oxygenation status of the tissue during IPoC which limits further interpretation. Nevertheless, the results suggest that for IPoC in the horse, the clamping cycle should be prolonged for consistent reduction in oxygenation. The approach might have to vary between species, taking differences in physiological heart rates and cardiac index into account. Furthermore, the location and technique of clamping may be relevant for the speed of de- and re-oxygenation. On the other hand, the exact mode of action of IPoC is still not clear, and it has been hypothesised that hypoxia may not be the key mediator for the induction of the protective mechanism (99). Should this indeed be the case, the pursuit of significant tissue oxygen desaturation would be futile.

Up to date, oxygenation and microperfusion have not been documented during intestinal IPC or IPoC. The only publication on microperfusion in relation to conditioning, is the report that showed IPC to significantly improve intestinal microvascular perfusion and tissue oxygenation at the end of reperfusion, measured by laser Doppler flowmetry (86). More research in this field is required to elucidate the role of blood flow reduction and hypoxia in IPC and IPoC.

9.2.3. Mucosal histomorphology

For studies investigating intestinal I/R injury, regardless of the species or model, mucosal histomorphology has generally been the main parameter to determine outcome. The original Chiu score for intestinal mucosal histomorphology following I/R injury included epithelial separation, haemorrhage and inflammatory cell infiltration, all put together within one score (13, 20). The intestinal samples from the current experimental studies showed varying degrees of haemorrhage which did not necessarily correlate with the degree of epithelial separation. Consequently, we introduced a separated Chiu score to facilitate an independent assessment of these features (22, 130). Furthermore, the severe haemorrhage in some of the sections obscured any potential inflammatory cells, complicating evaluation of the inflammatory component. Therefore, this component was removed from the score, and replaced by immunohistochemical staining for cytosolic calprotectin.

In both experimental trials, most ischaemia and reperfusion samples were assigned to grade 3 of the modified Chiu score. There is wide range in the extent of epithelial separation between a Chiu score of 2 and 4. This may result in lower sensitivity for more subtle differences. Therefore, a more sensitive morphometrical approach might be preferable and would allow to identify smaller, though still relevant differences in the extent of epithelial separation. This has been applied in several studies investigating I/R Injury in horses (108, 211) and was subsequently adapted for the IPoC study. Digitalisation of the slides enabled fast and reliable measurement. To avoid operator bias in the selection of the area of interest, this was started in the upper right corner of the screen and comprised the first 10 properly aligned subsequent villi. In slides with abundant aligned villi, a total number of 20 villi was assessed, however, this did not change the results.

9.2.4. Cell death

The loss of epithelial cells seen in the histological specimens may be the result of apoptosis or necrosis. Apoptosis, the programmed execution of cell death, is an important part of mucosal homeostasis due to the relatively short life span of epithelial cells (212). This mechanism can be upregulated in response to noxious stimuli or cell detachment from the basement membrane (213, 214). The caspase family, a group of cysteine proteases, are cellular proteins important for the initiation and execution of apoptosis (215). In the current study, we quantified the cells that stained positive for cleaved caspase-3, the active form of caspase 3, a downstream "executioner caspase" responsible for the cleavage of DNA fragmentation factor (216, 217). In our IPC study, a significant rise in cleaved caspase-3 positive cells was seen after 30 minutes of reperfusion. In enterocyte cell culture experiments, this caspase could be detected with immunohistochemistry within 30 - 45 minutes after detachment (218, 219). Comparing these time frames, it is possible that in our experiment the activation of the caspase cascade already took place during ischaemia. Interestingly, the cleaved caspase-3 cell counts in the IPoC study were only marginally higher, even though this experiment had a reperfusion duration of 120 minutes. This could indicate that there is no significant additional caspase activation during reperfusion in this experimental model.

We found that both xylazine PPC and IPoC resulted in lower cleaved caspase-3 counts. As a downstream caspase, the enzyme is activated by both the mitochondrial mediated intrinsic and the receptor mediated extrinsic pathway of the caspase cascade (216). Hence, the protective effect of PPC and IPoC could have been mediated through different intracellular pathways. Additional evaluation of the "initiator" caspases 2, 8, 9, and 10 could have yielded more information on the time frame and mode of activation (216, 219). For example, caspase-9 can be activated due to cessation of Akt-mediated phosphorylation (220), a feature that has been reported to play a role in both pre- and postconditioning (133, 139).

A TUNEL assay was also performed to assess the number of apoptotic cells. Originally, this assay was intended to identify cells in late apoptosis, because it detects double stranded DNA breaks. However, several studies have shown that TUNEL assays labelled both apoptotic and necrotic cells (221, 222), possibly due to more specific DNA degradation with double stranded DNA breaks during early necrosis (223). In the present study, the TUNEL positive cell counts were lower than their cleaved caspase-3 counterparts. DNA fragmentation has been observed 90 min after detachment and initiation of apoptosis (218), and therefore the caspase positive cells may not have reached this late stage of apoptosis during the time frame of the experiment.

A possible confounding factor in the quantification of the apoptotic and necrotic cells is that only cells that were still attached to the mucosa were included in the cell count. The cell debris in the intestinal lumen was not considered which could have led to an underestimation of apoptotic or necrotic cells in case of severe villus destruction. However, this approach was taken because the amount of cell debris was highly variable in the individual slides.

We also assessed the number of neurons in the myenteric plexus with ischaemia and reperfusion. To the author's knowledge, neuronal cell counts or intestinal motility measurements have so far not been investigated in IPC or IPoC. The neuron count per myenteric ganglion was highly variable at all time points, most likely affecting the analysis in this small sample size. Furthermore, the relatively short timeframe of reperfusion could have played a significant role, since previous studies have shown that neuronal apoptosis and loss does not occur before 6 and 24 hours of reperfusion, respectively (224-227). It is also possible that the damage to the intestine was not severe enough to induce neuronal cell death. Because the myenteric plexus was assessed on whole mount preparations, the submucosal plexus was not investigated, which may have responded sooner. However, this is not to be expected since previous studies have shown that the submucosal neurons are more resistant to ischaemia (224, 227). Moreover, neurons in the myenteric and submucosal plexus were not found to be TUNEL or cleaved caspase-3 positive which provides further evidence that neuronal damage does not occur within the first hours. This supports the finding that post-operative ileus in clinical cases usually develops after 12 - 24 hours (110, 228, 229). Both neuronal damage as well as the occurrence of post-operative ileus may be associated with the influx of neutrophils which is most pronounced around this time (227, 230, 231). The significance of enteric neuron damage in IPoC and equine post-ischaemic motility disorders remains unresolved, and future studies should take the requirement of prolonged reperfusion times into consideration.

9.2.5. Mucosal barrier function

The intestinal barrier function is vital because it prevents the invasion of toxins and bacteria from the intestinal lumen into the blood circulation. We found that the mucosal barrier function and nutrient absorption were significantly affected by ischaemia. The group subjected to IPoC had significantly lower mucosal to serosal fluxrates of mannitol, indicating that IPoC ameliorated the I/R induced increase in mucosal paracellular permeability. Experimental studies in rodents reported reduced bacterial translocation after both IPC and IPoC (87, 137), and IPC ameliorated intestinal hyperpermeability, as measured by the uptake of fluorescein labelled dextran (84). However, studies using the Ussing Chamber technique that would allow a comparison have not been performed.

Paracellular permeability is principally regulated by TJ proteins (232). In our IPoC study, the mucosal protein levels of claudin-1 and -2 as well as occludin were measured. The control group exhibited a significant decrease in all tested TJ protein levels at reperfusion compared to pre-ischaemia which could not be detected in group IPoC. This result may indicate that IPoC reduces the deterioration or increases the upregulation of TJ proteins. This could be mediated through a HIF response, since HIF-1α has been shown to regulate claudin-1 (176). The immunohistochemical HIF staining pattern observed in the current study does not support this theory, as there were no differences in HIF expression between the groups.

The expression and regulation of TJ proteins is also affected by cytokines such as TNF-α and interferon-γ (233-235). Neutrophils can either be a source of these cytokines, or cause direct damage through proteases or transmigration (200, 236). In the current study, we found no difference between the groups in mucosal inflammatory cell count to account for the difference in paracellular permeability. An alternative explanation for this decreased permeability would be that the smaller denuded epithelial surface area in group IPoC may have allowed less leakage compared to the more exposed lamina propria in the control group.

9.2.6. Inflammation

Most studies investigating IPC and IPoC looked at markers of inflammation, as the reduction of inflammation may be of significance for ameliorating I/R injury. In the current study, we assessed the local inflammation by counting the number of calprotectin positive cells in the different intestinal layers, and by measuring MPO in full thickness intestinal tissue. Both calprotectin and MPO are predominantly present in neutrophils, but are also expressed in monocytes and macrophages (237-239). There is a good correlation between neutrophils identified based on their morphology, and calprotectin-positive cells in the equine intestine

(231, 240), supporting the use of calprotectin as marker for neutrophilic infiltration. As in the previous conditioning studies, we only evaluated neutrophilic inflammation, because this is the most relevant leukocyte for acute ischaemic injury. The redistribution of mucosal eosinophils has been documented in the horse after naturally occurring strangulating obstructions; yet, this was not consistently observed in experimental jejunal ischaemia (241). Increased intestinal lymphoplasmacytic infiltration is predominantly associated with chronic inflammatory processes of stomach and intestines (242).

In both experimental studies, we found a significant increase in calprotectin positive cells after reperfusion. It has been suggested that the maximum neutrophil infiltration in horses occurs at a later stage, 12 - 24 hours after ischaemia (197, 231). Therefore, an extended period of reperfusion could have affected the result regarding the number and location of neutrophils. Nevertheless, we found a substantial increase in the neutrophil counts which has been shown to be associated with the occurrence of adhesions and post-operative ileus (12, 28-31). Even though the significance of mucosal reperfusion injury in the horse is under debate, most authors agree that the prevention of neutrophil infiltration in serosa and muscularis during reperfusion represents a potential therapeutic window to prevent postoperative complications (12, 37).

We found that preconditioning with xylazine reduced the neutrophil infiltration in both mucosa and serosa. Dexmedetomidine, another alpha-2-agonist, has also been associated with decreased inflammation, reducing the levels of lipid peroxidation (243, 244), hypoxanthine (243) and pro-inflammatory cytokines TNF-α and IL-6 (102, 245, 246). One study reported that these effects could be reversed of by the addition of alpha-2-antagonists, suggesting that the alpha-2 receptor mediates the anti-inflammatory effect of dexmedetomidine (247). Studies assessing this effect in xylazine are lacking; however, it is likely that its anti-inflammatory actions are mediated through the same pathway.

Lidocaine PPC did not affect the inflammatory cell count. In previous studies, the effect of lidocaine on intestinal inflammation in horses has been inconsistent. One group reported reduced mucosal neutrophil counts when treatment with flunixine-meglumine was combined with lidocaine administration (208), while another found no consistent decrease in neutrophil tissue infiltration (184). The exact response of inflammatory cells to lidocaine has not been clarified. It has been shown that lidocaine influences the function of neutrophil sodium channels in mice, thereby inhibiting their adhesion and migration (248). Furthermore, lidocaine decreased endotoxin-induced leukocyte-endothelial cell adhesion and macromolecular leakage in rats (249). In contrast, an in vitro experiment on equine neutrophils found that lidocaine did not inhibit neutrophil migration or adhesion at therapeutic concentrations and even increased migration and adhesion at higher concentrations (250). Considering the results of the various equine studies it has to be concluded that there is little evidence for an anti-inflammatory effect of lidocaine in the horse.

In our study investigating IPoC no treatment effect on neutrophilic inflammation was found. Considering that xylazine reduced inflammation in the PPC study, it must be noted that a single dose of xylazine was used in the premedication of the horses in the IPoC study. This could have elicited a PPC mediated anti-inflammatory effect, reducing the potential for this action by IPoC treatment. Nevertheless, xylazine was elected for premedication in this study because anaesthetic induction without prior sedation is associated with poor induction quality and concurrent animal welfare concerns, and there are no comparable alternatives without preconditioning effects. Of the available alpha-2-agonists, xylazine has the shortest duration of action (251). It has been suggested that the anti-inflammatory effects of dexmedetomidine are dose-dependent (247, 252). In the IPoC study, xylazine was administered in a lower dose compared to the PPC study, and it was not followed by a continuous rate infusion. Therefore, the preconditioning effect may not have been as potent as in the PPC study.

9.2.7. Mechanism of conditioning action in the current model

The studies investigating pre- and postconditioning in rodents have identified a multitude of different pathways that mediate the effect of conditioning. Nearly all published studies have reported a positive association between the pathway they were investigating and the effect of IPoC, making it difficult to rule out any mechanisms or pathways. This complicates the determination of the exact mechanism of conditioning, especially considering of the contradictory results that have been published by different research groups.

In our IPoC study, the parameters for inflammation and oxidative stress did not differ between the groups, indicating that IPoC protection is not mediated through the modulation of these presentations of I/R injury. We hypothesised that the heat shock response is of relevance for the mechanism underlying IPoC; however, the results of the HSP-70 immunohistochemistry study did not support this.

As mentioned before, different authors have linked both up- and downregulation of HIF-1α to the protective effect of pre- and postconditioning (129, 180, 253, 254). The current study did not detect any difference between the groups with regards to the expression of HIF-1α. Because this is only based on a semi-quantitative score, in combination with individual variation in staining pattern, a small sample size and a limited timeframe, it is possible that more subtle differences in immunoreactivity were overlooked. Hence, further quantitative analyses of HIF-1α expression and upregulation might allow more solid conclusions on its role in IPoC in horses. HIF-2α has not been previously assessed in the context of conditioning. Considering that we could not identify an effect of the ischaemia model on its expression, it is unlikely that HIF-2α would be of significance in the modulation of I/R injury by IPoC in the current model.

Both xylazine PPC and IPoC resulted in lower apoptotic cell counts, confirming the finding of many other experimental trials that conditioning elicits an anti-apoptotic effect. This is most likely conveyed by the activation of pro-survival kinases such as PI3K/Akt and ERK-1/2, (112, 171, 172) and the upregulation of anti-apoptotic regulators such as BCL-2 (75, 170, 172). However, we did not investigate these factors, and more research is needed to determine which triggers or receptors are responsible for the conditioning mediated protection in the horse.

9.2.8. The proximal intestinal segment

We know from previous studies that the intestinal segments peripheral to clinical intestinal ischaemia also show signs of damage and a stress response. The serosa at jejunal resection margins was shown to exhibit haemorrhage, oedema, and increased numbers of neutrophils (16). Furthermore, increased nuclear immunoreactivity for ubiquitin, HSP-70 and c-jun was seen at the oral border of clinical strangulating lesions (47).

In the IPoC study, an additional control sample was taken after reperfusion from the area 10 cm oral to the proximal luminal ligature. This area and time point was selected as a control for the effect of the surgical procedure without ischaemia, and to evaluate the response of the proximal segment to IPoC. This intestinal segment showed an increase in leukocyte infiltration after reperfusion in group IPoC only. This may be a consequence of prolonged exteriorisation or manipulation of the intestines during the postconditioning treatment. Because we found no difference in the direct comparison between the groups, the significance of this finding remains questionable. However, if this adverse effect would be confirmed by follow-up studies, it could represent a contraindication for the use of this postconditioning technique in clinical cases (12, 28-31).

The phenomenon of remote conditioning could have been applicable to the proximal segment of the horse intestine subjected to postconditioning. However, we could not detect significant remote injury, except for an increase in the serosal inflammatory cell count. Without significant I/R induced changes in this segment, it would not be possible to identify a significant protective effect of remote conditioning. Therefore, the current model and time-frame was found to be unsuitable to investigate the phenomenon of remote conditioning.

9.2.9. Limitations

Several limitations have been identified during the interpretation of the results, and most apply to both experimental studies. A main limitation of the study is the small sample size. Even though an a priori power analysis indicated sufficient power with this number of horses, a type 2 statistical error may have occurred due to the small sample size and biological variation. Nevertheless, entering more horses into the experiment would have meant that a higher number of animals had to be sacrificed. The study investigating PPC made use of a historical control group to limit the required number of horses. All aspects of the experiment were performed according to the same protocol and under guidance of those involved in the previous study. Therefore, we believe that the results of the historical group are comparable with the results of the test groups.

Another limitation of the study is that only the short-term effects of PPC and IPoC could be examined, with reperfusion times of 30 and 120 minutes, respectively. Within this time frame, the potential effect is limited to the early phase of protection when the upregulation of some proteins may not have occurred at this time point. Furthermore, long term survival and complications determine the efficacy of a treatment. Still, this experimental model does not allow a prolonged reperfusion time, because extended anaesthesia times in horses can compromise cardiovascular stability and induce muscular damage and inflammation. The alternative of subjecting the horses to recovery from anaesthesia prior to euthanasia was considered unethical.

All horses received isoflurane for the maintenance of general anaesthesia. Volatile anaesthetics have been shown to exhibit a preconditioning protective effect (105, 142). Therefore, the degree of mucosal injury might be reduced by isoflurane PPC across all groups, possibly making the detection of a treatment effect more difficult. In the preconditioning study, the mean isoflurane concentration of the control group was higher compared to the xylazine group, probably caused by the minimal alveolar concentration reducing properties of the latter. The protective effect of isoflurane has been shown to be dose dependent in cardiac ischaemia (105). Consequently, this higher isoflurane concentration in the control group may have levelled a PPC effect of the tested drugs. With hindsight it might have been preferable to maintain the isoflurane concentration of the different groups at the same level, as was done in the postconditioning experiment.

Histology and immunohistochemistry scoring was performed by only one observer, which could be considered a limitation. However, this is considered negligible, as the assessment was done in a blinded manner. Another possible source of bias could be the intestinal sampling sites. Samples were always taken from the same area and not in a random manner, possibly causing a site-dependent effect. On the other hand, this effect would have applied to all horses and could therefore not have interfered with the group comparison. Moreover, this ensures the comparability of the samples within one time point.

9.2.10 Practical applicability in a clinical setting

The occurrence of equine strangulating colic is unpredictable, thereby precluding the application of preconditioning before the ischaemic insult has commenced. Nevertheless, there may still be blood flow to the tissue in the early stages of ischaemia, presenting the opportunity to precondition the strangulated intestinal segment within the lesion prior to further damage. For the type of strangulating obstructions where increasingly more intestine is incorporated in the lesion over time, the surrounding intestinal segments may be preconditioned before their blood supply is affected. Furthermore, pre-stenotic and remote intestinal segments also sustain injury (16, 47, 184) that could benefit from a preconditioning effect. Therefore, there are several situations where the concept of preconditioning could be a feasible therapeutic strategy to reduce intestinal I/R Injury in colic horses.

The use of IPoC during colic surgery is feasible from a timing perspective. After manual resolution of the strangulating obstruction, the surgeon generally has access to the mesentery to apply some form of vessel re-occlusion. The occlusion with haemostatic clamps as performed in this experimental study, may be applied for short intestinal segments, yet it may be less suitable for a longer segment or for a very thick mesentery. A more practical option may be the manual re-occlusion of the vessels, or the release of ischaemia in a decelerated manner. Even though this study did not find damage to the mesentery following postconditioning, any manipulation of the mesentery must be performed carefully to avoid traumatic injury of the friable vessels.

9.3. Conclusions and future perspectives

Pharmacological preconditioning with the alpha-2-agonist xylazine in experimental small intestinal ischaemia in horses resulted in reduced apoptosis and inflammation. A concurrent reduction in mucosal histomorphological injury could not be found; therefore, the clinical significance of these findings remains uncertain. Preconditioning with lidocaine did not have any effect on the tested variables. These results support the use of xylazine in sedative analgesia and anaesthetic protocols for horses with strangulating small intestinal lesions. The timing of administration for this indication may be most appropriate in the timeframe between the diagnoses and surgical resolution of the lesion, or indicated for horses with a suspected strangulating obstruction that cannot undergo an exploratory laparotomy.

Ischaemic postconditioning by use of haemostatic forceps in the same experimental model resulted in effective reduction of blood flow during all clamping cycles. Still, the duration of the clamping cycle would need to be extended to establish significant desaturation in all cycles. The blood flow and saturation need to be investigated during different protocols and algorithms of IPoC, to determine the significance of these variables for the protective action of this treatment strategy. This would enable the determination of a more specific target for IPoC clamping, and consequently, it might be possible to calculate the optimal clamping sequence in relation to the size of the subject and the clamping method.

The intestinal mucosa of the horses subjected to IPoC demonstrated reduced villus denudation, para-cellular permeability and apoptosis rates compared to the untreated control group. This indicates a protective effect of IPoC on experimental intestinal I/R injury in horses. However, the exact mechanism of IPoC in the current model remains unclear. None of the other tested parameters were significantly affected by postconditioning, suggesting that the beneficial effects were not mediated by changes in inflammation, oxidative stress, heat shock response or hypoxia inducible factors. These negative results are in contradiction with the findings of many rodent studies investigating IPoC in small intestinal ischaemia. This disparity may be due to a difference in species, anaesthetic protocol, the applied ischaemia model and the degree of ischaemic injury. Furthermore, the small sample size and individual variability may have impaired the detection of smaller differences between the groups in the present study.

Even though there were no differences in HIF expression between the treatment groups, the HIF immunohistochemistry results have provided evidence to suggest that HIF-1α and not HIF-2α is of significance in the intestinal response to ischaemia. Furthermore, a distinct perinuclear HIF-2α staining pattern was associated with individual horses and not with the ischaemic event, which requires further investigation. More research including the quantitative analysis of HIF expression and their downstream targets would be necessary to determine the exact role of the HIF response in the equine intestine.

Both pharmacological preconditioning and ischaemic postconditioning hold potential for the treatment of mild to moderate intestinal I/R injury in equine colic cases. Before this can be implemented in patients, the long-term effects and the underlying protective mechanisms need to be determined. The development of in vitro models such as organoids would enable the investigation of potential mechanisms of action or further therapeutic strategies in addition to in vivo testing, reducing the need for animal experiments. Furthermore, clinical trials should be performed to assess the short- and long-term effects of conditioning in clinical cases of intestinal ischaemia.

10. References

1. Tinker MK, White N, Lessard P, Thatcher C, Pelzer K, Davis B, et al. Prospective study of equine colic incidence and mortality. Equine veterinary journal. 1997;29(6):448-53.
2. Archer D, Proudman C. Epidemiological clues to preventing colic. The Veterinary Journal. 2006;172(1):29-39.
3. Vachon AM, Fischer A. Small intestinal herniation through the epiploic foramen: 53 cases (1987–1993). Equine Veterinary Journal. 1995;27(5):373-80.
4. Huskamp B, editor The diagnosis and treatment of acute abdominal conditions in the horse; the various types and frequency as seen at the animal hospital in Hochmoor. Proceedings of the 1st Equine Colic Research Symposium; 1982.
5. Siebke A-U. Statistische Erhebung über Kurz-und Langzeitergebnisse von 718 operativ behandelten Kolikpatienten: na; 1995.
6. Phillips T, Walmsley J. Retrospective analysis of the results of 151 exploratory laparotomies in horses with gastrointestinal disease. Equine Veterinary Journal. 1993;25(5):427-31.
7. Freeman D, Hammock P, Baker G, Goetz T, Foreman JH, Schaeffer D, et al. Short-and long-term survival and prevalence of postoperative ileus after small intestinal surgery in the horse. Equine Veterinary Journal. 2000;32(S32):42-51.
8. Garcia-Seco E, Wilson DA, Kramer J, Keegan KG, Branson KR, Johnson PJ, et al. Prevalence and risk factors associated with outcome of surgical removal of pedunculated lipomas in horses: 102 cases (1987–2002). Journal of the American Veterinary Medical Association. 2005;226(9):1529-37.
9. Edwards G, Proudman C. An analysis of 75 cases of intestinal obstruction caused by pedunculated lipomas. Equine Veterinary Journal. 1994;26(1):18-21.
10. Stephen JO, Corley KT, Johnston JK, Pfeiffer D. Small intestinal volvulus in 115 horses: 1988–2000. Veterinary Surgery. 2004;33(4):333-9.
11. Auer JA, Stick JA, Kuemmerle JM, Prange T. Equine Surgery. 5th ed: Elsevier Health Sciences; 2019.
12. Blikslager AT. The Equine Acute Abdomen: John Wiley & Sons; 2017.
13. Chiu C-J, McArdle AH, Brown R, Scott HJ, Gurd FN. Intestinal mucosal lesion in low-flow states: I. A morphological, hemodynamic, and metabolic reappraisal. Archives of Surgery. 1970;101(4):478-83.
14. Dabareiner R, Snyder J, White N, Pascoe J, Harmon F, Gardner I, et al. Microvascular permeability and endothelial cell morphology associated with low-flow ischemia/reperfusion injury in the equine jejunum. American Journal of Veterinary Research. 1995;56(5):639-48.
15. Meschter C, Tyler D, White N, Moore J. Histologic findings in the gastrointestinal tract of horses with colic. American Journal of Veterinary Research. 1986;47(3):598-606.
16. Gerard M, Blikslager A, Roberts M, Tate Jr L, Argenzio R. The characteristics of intestinal injury peripheral to strangulating obstruction lesions in the equine small intestine. Equine Veterinary Journal. 1999;31(4):331-5.
17. Dart A, Snyder J, Julian D, Hinds D. Microvascular circulation of the small intestine in horses. American Journal of Veterinary Research. 1992;53(6):995.
18. Shepherd A, Granger DN. Metabolic regulation of the intestinal circulation. Physiology of the Intestinal Circulation. 1984:33-47.
19. Kalogeris T, Baines CP, Krenz M, Korthuis RJ. Chapter Six - Cell Biology of Ischemia/Reperfusion Injury. In: Jeon KW, editor. International Review of Cell and Molecular Biology. 298: Academic Press; 2012. p. 229-317.
20. White N, Moore J, Trim C. Mucosal alterations in experimentally induced small intestinal strangulation obstruction in ponies. American Journal of Veterinary Research. 1980;41(2):193-8.
21. Dabareiner RM, Sullins KE, White NA, Snyder JR. Serosal injury in the equine jejunum and ascending colon after ischemia-reperfusion or intraluminal distention and decompression. Veterinary Surgery. 2001;30(2):114-25.
22. Gonzalez LM, Fogle CA, Baker WT, Hughes FE, Law JM, Motsinger-Reif AA, et al. Operative factors associated with short-term outcome in horses with large colon volvulus: 47 cases from 2006 to 2013. Equine Veterinary Journal 2015;47(3):279-84.
23. Park P, Haglund U, Bulkley G, Fält K. The sequence of development of intestinal tissue injury after strangulation ischemia and reperfusion. Surgery. 1990;107(5):574-80.

24. Laws EG, Freeman DE. Significance of reperfusion injury after venous strangulation obstruction of equine jejunum. Journal of Investigative Surgery. 1995;8(4):263-70.
25. Prichard M, Ducharme NG, Wilkins PA, Erb HN, Butt M. Xanthine oxidase formation during experimental ischemia of the equine small intestine. Canadian Journal of Veterinary Research. 1991;55(4):310.
26. Granger DN, Parks DA. Role of oxygen radicals in the pathogenesis of intestinal ischemia. The Physiologist. 1983;26(3):159-64.
27. Johnston J, Freeman D, Gillette D, Soma L. Effects of superoxide dismutase on injury induced by anoxia and reoxygenation in equine small intestine in vitro. American Journal of Veterinary Research. 1991;52(12):2050-4.
28. Bodi N, Szalai Z, Bagyanszki M. Nitrergic Enteric Neurons in Health and Disease-Focus on Animal Models. Int J Mol Sci. 2019;20(8).
29. Lundin C, Sullins K, White N, Clem M, Debowes R, Pfeiffer C. Induction of peritoneal adhesions with small intestinal ischaemia and distention in the foal. Equine Veterinary Journal. 1989;21(6):451-8.
30. Lisowski ZM, Pirie RS, Blikslager AT, Lefebvre D, Hume DA, Hudson NPH. An update on equine post-operative ileus: Definitions, pathophysiology and management. Equine Veterinary Journal 2018;50(3):292-303.
31. Türler A, Kalff JC, Moore BA, Hoffman RA, Billiar TR, Simmons RL, et al. Leukocyte-derived inducible nitric oxide synthase mediates murine postoperative ileus. Annals of Surgery. 2006;244(2):220.
32. Vatistas NJ, Snyder JR, Hildebrand S, Harmon FA, Woliner MJ, Barry SJ, et al. Effects of U-74389G, a novel 21-aminosteroid, on small intestinal ischemia and reperfusion injury in horses. American Journal of Veterinary Research. 1996;57(5):762-70.
33. Freeman DE, Schaeffer DJ, Baker GJ, editors. A Clinical Grading System for Intraoperative Assessment of Small Intestinal Viability in the Horse. AAEP Proceedings Vol 47; 2001.
34. Freeman DE, Gentile DG, Richardson DW, Fetrow JP, Tulleners EP, Orsini JA, et al. Comparison of clinical judgment, Doppler ultrasound, and fluorescein fluorescence as methods for predicting intestinal viability in the pony. American Journal of Veterinary Research. 1988;49(6):895-900.
35. Snyder J, Pascoe J, Holland M, Kurpershoek C. Surface oximetry of healthy and ischemic equine intestine. American Journal of Veterinary Research. 1986;47(12):2530-5.
36. Van Hoogmoed L, Snyder JR, Pascoe JR, Olander H. Use of pelvic flexure biopsies to predict survival after large colon torsion in horses. Veterinary Surgery. 2000;29(6):572-7.
37. Auer JA, Stick JA, Kuemmerle JM, Prange T. Equine Surgery. 5 ed. St. Louis, Missouri: Elsevier; 2019.
38. MacDonald MH, Pascoe JR, Stover SM, Meagher DM. Survival after small intestine resection and anastomosis in horses. Veterinary Surgery. 1990;18(6):415-23.
39. Close K, Epstein KL, Sherlock CE. A retrospective study comparing the outcome of horses undergoing small intestinal resection and anastomosis with a single layer (Lembert) or double layer (simple continuous and Cushing) technique. Veterinary Surgery. 2014;43(4):471-8.
40. Stephen JO, Corley KT, Johnston JK, Pfeiffer D. Factors associated with mortality and morbidity in small intestinal volvulus in horses. Veterinary Surgery. 2004;33(4):340-8.
41. Proudman C, Edwards G, Barnes J, French N. Factors affecting long-term survival of horses recovering from surgery of the small intestine. Equine Veterinary Journal. 2005;37(4):360-5.
42. Mair T, Smith L. Survival and complication rates in 300 horses undergoing surgical treatment of colic. Part 1: short-term survival following a single laparotomy. Equine Veterinary Journal. 2005;37(4):296-302.
43. Freeman DE, Schaeffer DJ, Cleary OB. Long-term survival in horses with strangulating obstruction of the small intestine managed without resection. Equine Veterinary Journal. 2014;46(6):711-7.
44. Kersjes A, Bras G, Nemeth F, Van der Velden M, Firth E. Results of operative treatment of equine colic with special reference to surgery of the ileum. Veterinary Quarterly. 1988;10(1):17-25.
45. Tate Jr L, Ralston S, Koch C, Everitt J. Effects of extensive resection of the small intestine in the pony. American Journal of Veterinary Research. 1983;44(7):1187-91.
46. Haven M, Roberts M, Argenzio R, Bowman K, Meuten D, editors. Intestinal adaptation following 70% small bowel resection in ponies. Proceedings of the 4th Equine Colic Research Symposium; 1991.
47. De Ceulaer K, Delesalle C, Van Elzen R, Van Brantegem L, Weyns A, Van Ginneken C. Morphological data indicate a stress response at the oral border of strangulated small intestine in horses. Research in Veterinary Science. 2011;91(2):294-300.
48. Parker JE, Fubini SL, Todhunter RJ. Retrospective evaluation of repeat celiotomy in 53 horses with acute gastrointestinal disease. Veterinary Surgery. 1990;18(6):424-31.

49. Horne MM, Pascoe PJ, Ducharme NG, Barker IK, Grovum WL. Attempts to modify reperfusion injury of equine jejunal mucosa using dimethylsulfoxide, allopurinol, and intraluminal oxygen. Veterinary Surgery. 1994;23(4):241-9.
50. Hoogmoed LMV, Nieto JE, Spier SJ, Snyder JR. In vivo investigation of the efficacy of a customized solution to attenuate injury following low-flow ischemia and reperfusion injury in the jejunum of horses. American Journal of Veterinary Research. 2004;65(4):485-90.
51. Dabareiner R, II NW, Donaldson L. Evaluation of Carolina Rinse solution as a treatment for ischaemia reperfusion of the equine jejunum. Equine Veterinary Journal. 2003;35(7):642-6.
52. Rötting AK, Freeman DE, Eurell JAC, Constable PD, Wallig M. Effects of acetylcysteine and migration of resident eosinophils in an in vitro model of mucosal injury and restitution in equine right dorsal colon. American Journal of Veterinary Research. 2003;64(10):1205-12.
53. Cook V, Shults JJ, McDowell M, Campbell N, Davis J, Blikslager A. Attenuation of ischaemic injury in the equine jejunum by administration of systemic lidocaine. Equine Veterinary Journal. 2008;40(4):353-7.
54. Moore R, Bertone A, Muir W. Effect of high-molecular weight dextran macromolecules on low-flow ischemia and reperfusion of the large colon in horses. American Journal of Veterinary Research. 1996;57(7):1067-73.
55. Moore RM, Muir WW, Bertone AL, Oliver JL. Effect of Platelet-Activating Factor Antagonist L-691,880 on Low-Flow Ischemia-Reperfusion Injury of the Large Colon in Horses. Veterinary Surgery. 1998;27(1):37-48.
56. Gupta R, Wood DA. Primary prevention of ischaemic heart disease: populations, individuals, and health professionals. The Lancet. 2019;394(10199):685-96.
57. Mattson MP. Hormesis defined. Ageing Research Reviews. 2008;7(1):1-7.
58. Murry CE, Jennings RB, Reimer KA. Preconditioning with ischemia: a delay of lethal cell injury in ischemic myocardium. Circulation. 1986;74(5):1124-36.
59. Nakamura M, Wang N-P, Zhao Z-Q, Wilcox JN, Thourani V, Guyton RA, et al. Preconditioning decreases Bax expression, PMN accumulation and apoptosis in reperfused rat heart. Cardiovascular Research. 2000;45(3):661-70.
60. Richard V, Kaeffer N, Tron C, Thuillez C. Myocardial ischemia/reperfusion/PTCA: ischemic preconditioning protects against coronary endothelial dysfunction induced by ischemia and reperfusion. Circulation. 1994;89:1254-61.
61. DeFily DV, Chilian WM. Preconditioning protects coronary arteriolar endothelium from ischemia-reperfusion injury. American Journal of Physiology-Heart and Circulatory Physiology. 1993;265(2):H700-H6.
62. Piot CA, Padmanaban D, Ursell PC, Sievers RE, Wolfe CL. Ischemic preconditioning decreases apoptosis in rat hearts in vivo. Circulation. 1997;96(5):1598-604.
63. Lott FD, Guo P, Toombs CF. Reduction in infarct size by ischemic preconditioning persists in a chronic rat model of myocardial ischemia-reperfusion injury. Pharmacology. 1996;52(2):113-8.
64. Jebeli M, Esmaili HR, Mandegar MH, Rasouli MR, Eghtesadi-Araghi P, Mohammadzadeh R, et al. Evaluation of the effects of ischemic preconditioning with a short reperfusion phase on patients undergoing a coronary artery bypass graft. Annals of Thoracic and Cardiovascular Surgery 2010;16(4):248-52.
65. Wu Z-k, Tarkka MR, Eloranta J, Pehkonen E, Kaukinen L, Honkonen EL, et al. Effect of ischemic preconditioning on myocardial protection in coronary artery bypass graft patients: can the free radicals act as a trigger for ischemic preconditioning? Chest. 2001;119(4):1061-8.
66. Jenkins DP, Pugsley WB, Alkhulaifi AM, Kemp M, Hooper J, Yellon DM. Ischaemic preconditioning reduces troponin T release in patients undergoing coronary artery bypass surgery. Heart. 1997;77(4):314-8.
67. Kaukoranta PK, Lepojärvi MP, Ylitalo KV, Kiviluoma KT, Peuhkurinen KJ. Normothermic retrograde blood cardioplegia with or without preceding ischemic preconditioning. The Annals of Thoracic Surgery. 1997;63(5):1268-74.
68. Cremer J, Steinhoff G, Karck M, Ahnsell T, Brandt M, Teebken O, et al. Ischemic preconditioning prior to myocardial protection with cold blood cardioplegia in coronary surgery. European Journal of Cardio-thoracic Surgery. 1997;12(5):753-8.
69. Lee W-Y, Lee S-M. Ischemic preconditioning protects post-ischemic oxidative damage to mitochondria in rat liver. Shock. 2005;24(4):370-5.

70. Hasegawa T, Malle E, Farhood A, Jaeschke H. Generation of hypochlorite-modified proteins by neutrophils during ischemia-reperfusion injury in rat liver: attenuation by ischemic preconditioning. American Journal of Physiology-Gastrointestinal and Liver Physiology. 2005;289(4):G760-G7.
71. Clavien P-A, Selzner M, Rüdiger HA, Graf R, Kadry Z, Rousson V, et al. A prospective randomized study in 100 consecutive patients undergoing major liver resection with versus without ischemic preconditioning. Annals of Surgery. 2003;238(6):843.
72. Weiwei Chu SL, Shanwei Wang, Aili Yan, Lei Nie. Ischemic postconditioning provides protection against ischemia-reperfusion injury in intestines of rats. International Journal of Clinical and Experimental Pathology. 2015;8(6):6474 - 81.
73. Juel IS, Solligård E, Tvedt KE, Skogvoll E, Jynge P, Beisvag V, et al. Post-ischaemic restituted intestinal mucosa is more resistant to further ischaemia than normal mucosa in the pig. Scandinavian Journal of Clinical and Laboratory Investigation. 2008;68(2):106-16.
74. Santos CH, Gomes OM, Pontes JC, Miiji LN, Bispo MA. The ischemic preconditioning and postconditioning effect on the intestinal mucosa of rats undergoing mesenteric ischemia/reperfusion procedure. Acta Cirurgica Brasileira / Sociedade Brasileira para Desenvolvimento Pesquisa em Cirurgia. 2008;23(1):22-8.
75. Cinel I, Avlan D, Cinel L, Polat G, Atici S, Mavioglu I, et al. Ischemic preconditioning reduces intestinal epithelial apoptosis in rats. Shock. 2003;19(6):588-92.
76. Unal S, Demirkan F, Arslan E, Cin I, Cinel L, Eskandari G, et al. Comparison of Ischemic and Chemical Preconditioning in Jejunal Flaps in the Rat. Plastic and Reconstructive Surgery. 2003;112(4):1024-31.
77. Zhang Y, Wu Y-X, Hao Y-B, Dun Y, Yang S-P. Role of endogenous opioid peptides in protection of ischemic preconditioning in rat small intestine. Life Sciences. 2001;68(9):1013-9.
78. Moore-Olufemi SD, Kozar RA, Moore FA, Sato N, Hassoun HT, Cox CSJ, et al. Ischemic preconditioning protects against gut dysfunction and mucosal injury after ischemia/reperfusion injury. Shock. 2005;23(3):258-63.
79. Jacome DT, Abrahao MS, Morello RJ, Martins JL, Medeiros AC, Montero EF. Different intervals of ischemic preconditioning on small bowel ischemia-reperfusion injury in rats. Transplant Proceedings. 2009;41(3):827-9.
80. Varga J, Tóth Š, Staško P, Bujdoš M, Veselá J, Jonecová Z, et al. Different ischemic preconditioning regimens affecting preservation injury of intestines. European Surgical Research. 2011;46(4):207-13.
81. Aufricht C, Bidmon B, Ruffingshofer D, Regele H, Herkner K, Siegel NJ, et al. Ischemic conditioning prevents Na,K-ATPase dissociation from the cytoskeletal cellular fraction after repeat renal ischemia in rats. Pediatric Research. 2002;51(6):722-7.
82. Tamion F, Richard V, Lacoume Y, Thuillez C. Intestinal preconditioning prevents systemic inflammatory response in hemorrhagic shock. Role of HO-1. American journal of Physiology Gastrointestinal and liver Physiology. 2002;283(2):G408-14.
83. Erling Junior N, Montero EFdS, Sannomiya P, Poli-de-Figueiredo LF. Local and remote ischemic preconditioning protect against intestinal ischemic/reperfusion injury after supraceliac aortic clamping. Clinics. 2013;68(12):1548-54.
84. McCallion K, Wattanasirichaigoon S, Gardiner KR, Fink MP. Ischemic preconditioning ameliorates ischemia-and reperfusion-induced intestinal epithelial hyperpermeability in rats. Shock. 2000;14(4):429-34.
85. Yang S-P, Hao Y, Wu Y-X, Dun W, Shen L-H, Zhang Y. Ischemic preconditioning mediated by activation of KATP channels in rat small intestine. Zhongguo yao li xue bao= Acta Pharmacologica Sinica. 1999;20(4):341-4.
86. Mallick I, Yang W, Winslet M, Seifalian A. Ischaemic preconditioning improves microvascular perfusion and oxygenation following reperfusion injury of the intestine. British Journal of Surgery. 2005;92(9):1169-76.
87. Aksöyek S, Cinel I, Avlan D, Cinel L, Öztürk C, Gürbüz P, et al. Intestinal ischemic preconditioning protects the intestine and reduces bacterial translocation. Shock. 2002;18(5):476-80.
88. Wu B, Ootani A, Iwakiri R, Fujise T, Tsunada S, Toda S, et al. Ischemic preconditioning attenuates ischemia-reperfusion-induced mucosal apoptosis by inhibiting the mitochondria-dependent pathway in rat small intestine. American Journal of Physiology-Gastrointestinal and Liver Physiology. 2004;286(4):G580-G7.
89. Hotter G, Closa D, Prados M, Fernández-Cruz L, Prats N, Gelpı E, et al. Intestinal preconditioning is mediated by a transient increase in nitric oxide. Biochemical and Biophysical Research Communications. 1996;222(1):27-32.

90. Sola A, Hotter G, Prats N, Xaus C, Gelpí E, Roselló-Catafau J. Modification of oxidative stress in response to intestinal preconditioning1. Transplantation. 2000;69(5):767-72.
91. Mallick IH, Winslet MC, Seifalian AM. Ischemic preconditioning of small bowel mitigates the late phase of reperfusion injury: heme oxygenase mediates cytoprotection. The American Journal of Surgery. 2010;199(2):223-31.
92. Saeki I, Matsuura T, Hayashida M, Taguchi T. Ischemic preconditioning and remote ischemic preconditioning have protective effect against cold ischemia–reperfusion injury of rat small intestine. Pediatric Surgery International. 2011;27(8):857-62.
93. Sola A, De Oca J, González R, Prats N, Roselló-Catafau J, Gelpí E, et al. Protective effect of ischemic preconditioning on cold preservation and reperfusion injury associated with rat intestinal transplantation. Annals of Surgery. 2001;234(1):98.
94. Wang S-F, Li G-W. Early protective effect of ischemic preconditioning on small intestinal graft in rats. World Journal of Gastroenterology. 2003;9(8):1866.
95. Ferencz A, Szántó Z, Borsiczky B, Kiss K, Kalmár-Nagy K, Szeberényi J, et al. The effects of preconditioning on the oxidative stress in small-bowel autotransplantation. Surgery. 2002;132(5):877-84.
96. Ferencz A, Szanto Z, Kalmar-Nagy K, Horváth ÖP, Roth E, editors. Mitigation of oxidative injury by classic and delayed ischemic preconditioning prior to small bowel autotransplantation. Transplantation Proceedings; 2004: Elsevier.
97. König KS, Verhaar N, Hopster K, Pfarrer C, Neudeck S, Rohn K, et al. Ischaemic preconditioning and pharmacological preconditioning with dexmedetomidine in an equine model of small intestinal ischaemia-reperfusion. PlOS ONE. 2020;15(4):e0224720.
98. Gross ER, Gross GJ. Ligand triggers of classical preconditioning and postconditioning. Cardiovascular Research. 2006;70(2):212-21.
99. Krenz M, Baines C, Kalogeris T, Korthuis R, editors. Cell survival programs and ischemia/reperfusion: hormesis, preconditioning, and cardioprotection. Colloquium Series on Integrated Systems Physiology: From Molecule to Function to Disease; 2013: Morgan & Claypool Life Sciences.
100. Dun Y, Hao Y-B, Wu Y-X, Zhang Y, Zhao R-R. Protective effects of nitroglycerin-induced preconditioning mediated by calcitonin gene-related peptide in rat small intestine. European Journal of Pharmacology. 2001;430(2-3):317-24.
101. Liu C, Shen Z, Liu Y, Peng J, Miao L, Zeng W, et al. Sevoflurane protects against intestinal ischemia-reperfusion injury partly by phosphatidylinositol 3 kinases/Akt pathway in rats. Surgery. 2015;157(5):924-33.
102. Sun Y, Gao Q, Wu N, Li SD, Yao JX, Fan WJ. Protective effects of dexmedetomidine on intestinal ischemia-reperfusion injury. Experimental and Therapeutic Medicine. 2015;10(2):647-52.
103. Sayan H, Ozacmak VH, Sen F, Cabuk M, Atik DY, Igdem AA, et al. Pharmacological preconditioning with erythropoietin reduces ischemia–reperfusion injury in the small intestine of rats. Life Sciences. 2009;84(11-12):364-71.
104. Zhao B, Fei J, Chen Y, Ying Y-L, Ma L, Song X-Q, et al. Pharmacological preconditioning with vitamin C attenuates intestinal injury via the induction of heme oxygenase-1 after hemorrhagic shock in rats. PLOS ONE. 2014;9(6):e99134.
105. Zhang L, Huang H, Cheng J, Liu J, Zhao H, Vizcaychipi MP, et al. Pre-treatment with isoflurane ameliorates renal ischemic-reperfusion injury in mice. Life Sciences. 2011;88(25-26):1102-7.
106. Kostopanagiotou G, Avgerinos ED, Markidou E, Voiniadis P, Chondros C, Theodoraki K, et al. Protective effect of NAC preconditioning against ischemia-reperfusion injury in piglet small bowel transplantation: effects on plasma TNF, IL-8, hyaluronic acid, and NO. Journal of Surgical Research. 2011;168(2):301-5.
107. Kılıç K, Hancı V, Selek Ş, Sözmen M, Kiliç N, Çitil M, et al. The effects of dexmedetomidine on mesenteric arterial occlusion-associated gut ischemia and reperfusion-induced gut and kidney injury in rabbits. Journal of Surgical Research. 2012;178(1):223-32.
108. VanderBroek AR, Engiles JB, Kästner SB, Kopp V, Verhaar N, Hopster K. Protective effects of dexmedetomidine on small intestinal ischaemia-reperfusion injury in horses. Equine Veterinary Journal. 2020.
109. Rezende M, Grimsrud KN, Stanley SD, Steffey E, Mama K. Pharmacokinetics and pharmacodynamics of intravenous dexmedetomidine in the horse. Journal of Veterinary Pharmacology and Therapeutics. 2015;38(1):15-23.
110. Lefebvre D, Pirie R, Handel I, Tremaine W, Hudson N. Clinical features and management of equine post operative ileus: Survey of diplomates of the E uropean C olleges of E quine I nternal M edicine (ECEIM) and V eterinary S urgeons (ECVS). Equine Veterinary Journal. 2016;48(2):182-7.

111. Zhi-Qing Zhao JSC, Michael E. Halkos, Faraz Kerendi,, Ning-Ping Wang RAG, and Jakob Vinten-Johansen. Inhibition of myocardial injury by ischemic postconditioning during reperfusion: comparison with ischemic preconditioning. The American Journal of Physiology - Heart and Circulatory Physiology. 2003;285:579-88.
112. Hausenloy DJ, Tsang A, Mocanu MM, Yellon DM. Ischemic preconditioning protects by activating prosurvival kinases at reperfusion. The American Journal of Physiology - Heart and Circulatory Physiology. 2005;288(2):H971-H6.
113. Galagudza M, Kurapeev D, Minasian S, Valen G, Vaage J. Ischemic postconditioning: brief ischemia during reperfusion converts persistent ventricular fibrillation into regular rhythm. European Journal of Cardio-thoracic Surgery. 2004;25(6):1006-10.
114. Wagner C, Ebner B, Tillack D, Strasser RH, Weinbrenner C. Cardioprotection by ischemic postconditioning is abrogated in hypertrophied myocardium of spontaneously hypertensive rats. Journal of Cardiovascular Pharmacology. 2013;61(1):35-41.
115. Zhang L, Ma J, Liu H. Protective effect of ischemic postconditioning against ischemia reperfusion-induced myocardium oxidative injury in IR rats. Molecules. 2012;17(4):3805-17.
116. Lønborg J, Kelbæk H, Vejlstrup N, Jørgensen E, Helqvist S, Saunamäki K, et al. Cardioprotective effects of ischemic postconditioning in patients treated with primary percutaneous coronary intervention, evaluated by magnetic resonance. Circulation: Cardiovascular Interventions. 2010;3(1):34-41.
117. Ivanes F, Rioufol G, Piot C, Ovize M. Postconditioning in acute myocardial infarction patients. Antioxidants & Redox Signaling. 2011;14(5):811-20.
118. Lou B, Cui Y, Gao H, Chen M. Meta-analysis of the effects of ischemic postconditioning on structural pathology in ST-segment elevation acute myocardial infarction. Oncotarget. 2018;9(8):8089.
119. Kontis E, Pantiora E, Melemeni A, Tsaroucha A, Karvouni E, Polydorou A, et al. Ischemic postconditioning decreases iNOS gene expression but ischemic preconditioning ameliorates histological injury in a swine model of extended liver resection. Translational Gastroenterology and Hepatology. 2019;4.
120. Tian Y, Shu J, Huang R, Chu X, Mei X. Protective effect of renal ischemic postconditioning in renal ischemic-reperfusion injury. Translational Andrology and Urology. 2020;9(3):1356.
121. Wang J-y, Shen J, Gao Q, Ye Z-g, Yang S-y, Liang H-w, et al. Ischemic postconditioning protects against global cerebral ischemia/reperfusion-induced injury in rats. Stroke. 2008;39(3):983-90.
122. Xu B, Gao X, Xu J, Lei S, Xia Z-y, Xu Y, et al. Ischemic postconditioning attenuates lung reperfusion injury and reduces systemic proinflammatory cytokine release via heme oxygenase 1. Journal of Surgical Research. 2011;166(2):e157-e64.
123. Song W, Sun J, Su B, Yang R, Dong H, Xiong L. Ischemic postconditioning protects the spinal cord from ischemia–reperfusion injury via modulation of redox signaling. The Journal of Thoracic and Cardiovascular Surgery. 2013;146(3):688-95.
124. Minutoli L, Irrera N, Squadrito F, Marini H, Nicotina P, Arena S, et al. Effects of ischaemic post-conditioning on the early and late testicular damage after experimental testis ischaemia–reperfusion. Andrology. 2014;2(1):76-82.
125. Santos CHMd, Dourado DM, Sampaio TL, Dias LdES, Almeida MHMd, Oliva JVDG, et al. Effect of postconditioning and atorvastatin in preventing remote intestinal reperfusion injury. Journal of Coloproctology. 2017;37(4):301-5.
126. Liu KX, Li YS, Huang WQ, Chen SQ, Wang ZX, Liu JX, et al. Immediate postconditioning during reperfusion attenuates intestinal injury. Intensive Care Medicine 2009;35(5):933-42.
127. Cheng C-H, Lin H-C, Lai IR, Lai H-S. Ischemic postconditioning attenuate reperfusion injury of small intestine: impact of mitochondrial permeability transition. Transplantation. 2013;95(4):559-65.
128. Wen SH, Ling YH, Li Y, Li C, Liu JX, Li YS, et al. Ischemic postconditioning during reperfusion attenuates oxidative stress and intestinal mucosal apoptosis induced by intestinal ischemia/reperfusion via aldose reductase. Surgery. 2013;153(4):555-64.
129. Jia Z, Lian W, Shi H, Cao C, Han S, Wang K, et al. Ischemic Postconditioning Protects Against Intestinal Ischemia/Reperfusion Injury via the HIF-1alpha/miR-21 Axis. Scientific Reports. 2017;7(1):16190.
130. Sengul I, Sengul D, Guler O, Hasanoglu A, Urhan MK, Taner AS, et al. Postconditioning attenuates acute intestinal ischemia-reperfusion injury. The Kaohsiung Journal of Medical Sciences. 2013;29(3):119-27.
131. Rosero O, Onody P, Stangl R, Turoczi Z, Fulop A, Garbaisz D, et al. Postconditioning of the small intestine: which is the most effective algorithm in a rat model? Journal of Surgical Research. 2014;187(2):427-37.
132. Li YS, Wang ZX, Li C, Xu M, Li Y, Huang WQ, et al. Proteomics of ischemia/reperfusion injury in rat intestine with and without ischemic postconditioning. Journal of Surgical Research. 2010;164(1):e173-80.

133. Chen R, Zhang Y-y, Lan J-n, Liu H-m, Li W, Wu Y, et al. Ischemic Postconditioning Alleviates Intestinal Ischemia-Reperfusion Injury by Enhancing Autophagy and Suppressing Oxidative Stress through the Akt/GSK-3β/Nrf2 Pathway in Mice. Oxidative Medicine and Cellular Longevity. 2020;2020.
134. Ozkisacik S, Erdem AO, Etensel B, Tataroglu C, Serter M, Yazici M. Short-interval postconditioning protects the bowel against ischaemia-reperfusion injury in rats. Journal of International Medical Research. 2017;45(3):1036-41.
135. Santos CH, Aydos RD, Nogueira Neto E, Miiji LN, Cassino PC, Ahmed, II, et al. Importance of duration and number of ischemic postconditioning cycles in preventing reperfusion mesenteric injuries. Experimental study in rats. Acta Cirúrgica Brasileira. 2015;30(10):709-14.
136. Wen SH, Li Y, Li C, Xia ZQ, Liu WF, Zhang XY, et al. Ischemic postconditioning during reperfusion attenuates intestinal injury and mucosal cell apoptosis by inhibiting JAK/STAT signaling activation. Shock. 2012;38(4):411-9.
137. Rosero O, Onody P, Kovacs T, Molnar D, Lotz G, Toth S, et al. Impaired intestinal mucosal barrier upon ischemia-reperfusion: "patching holes in the shield with a simple surgical method". Biomed Research International. 2014;2014:210901.
138. Feng D, Li Z, Wang G, Yao J, Li Y, Qasim W, et al. Microarray Analysis of Differentially Expressed Profiles of Circular RNAs in a Mouse Model of Intestinal Ischemia/Reperfusion Injury with and Without Ischemic Postconditioning. Cell Physiol Biochem. 2018;48(4):1579-94.
139. Chen R, Zeng Z, Zhang Yy, Cao C, Liu Hm, Li W, et al. Ischemic postconditioning attenuates acute kidney injury following intestinal ischemia-reperfusion through Nrf2-regulated autophagy, anti-oxidation, and anti-inflammation in mice. The FASEB Journal. 2020.
140. Bretz B, Blaze C, Parry N, Kudej RK. Ischemic postconditioning does not attenuate ischemia-reperfusion injury of rabbit small intestine. Veterinary Surgery. 2010;39(2):216-23.
141. Ferencz A, Takacs I, Horvath S, Ferencz S, Javor S, Fekecs T, et al. Examination of protective effect of ischemic postconditioning after small bowel autotransplantation. Transplantation Proceedings. 2010;42(6):2287-9.
142. Albrecht M, Gruenewald M, Zitta K, Zacharowski K, Scholz J, Bein B, et al. Hypothermia and anesthetic postconditioning influence the expression and activity of small intestinal proteins possibly involved in ischemia/reperfusion-mediated events following cardiopulmonary resuscitation. Resuscitation. 2012;83(1):113-8.
143. Li Q, Cui S, Jing G, Ding H, Xia Z, He X. The role of PI3K/Akt signal pathway in the protective effects of propofol on intestinal and lung injury induced by intestinal ischemia/reperfusion. Acta cirurgica brasileira. 2019;34(1).
144. Burley DS, Baxter GF. Pharmacological targets revealed by myocardial postconditioning. Current Opinion in Pharmacology. 2009;9(2):177-88.
145. Kharbanda R, Mortensen U, White P, Kristiansen S, Schmidt M, Hoschtitzky J, et al. Transient limb ischemia induces remote ischemic preconditioning in vivo. Circulation. 2002;106(23):2881-3.
146. Kerendi F, Kin H, Halkos M, Jiang R, Zatta A, Zhao Z, et al. Brief renal ischemia and reperfusion applied before coronary artery reperfusion reduces myocardial infarct size via endogenous activation of adenosine receptors. Basic Research in Cardiology. 2005;100(5):404-12.
147. Sun X-C, Xian X-H, Li W-B, Li L, Yan C-Z, Li Q-J, et al. Activation of p38 MAPK participates in brain ischemic tolerance induced by limb ischemic preconditioning by up-regulating HSP 70. Experimental Neurology. 2010;224(2):347-55.
148. Selimoglu O, Ugurlucan M, Basaran M, Gungor F, Banach M, Cucu O, et al. Efficacy of remote ischaemic preconditioning for spinal cord protection against ischaemic injury: association with heat shock protein expression. Folia Neuropathology 2008;46(3):204-12.
149. Leng YF, Zhang Y, Zhang Y, Xue X, Wang T, Kang YQ. Ischemic post-conditioning attenuates the intestinal injury induced by limb ischemia/reperfusion in rats. Brazilian Journal of Medical and Biological Research. 2011;44(5):411-7.
150. Turoczi Z, Fulop A, Czigany Z, Varga G, Rosero O, Tokes T, et al. Improvement of small intestinal microcirculation by postconditioning after lower limb ischemia. Microvasc Res. 2015;98:119-25.
151. Ates E, Genç E, Erkasap N, Erkasap S, Akman S, Firat P, et al. Renal protection by brief liver ischemia in rats1. Transplantation. 2002;74(9):1247-51.
152. Walsh M, Whitlock R, Garg AX, Légaré J-F, Duncan AE, Zimmerman R, et al. Effects of remote ischemic preconditioning in high-risk patients undergoing cardiac surgery (Remote IMPACT): a randomized controlled trial. The Canadian Medical Association Journal. 2016;188(5):329-36.

153. Liu Z, Wang Y-L, Xu D, Hua Q, Chu Y-Y, Ji X-M. Late remote ischemic preconditioning provides benefit to patients undergoing elective percutaneous coronary intervention. Cell Biochemistry and Biophysics. 2014;70(1):437-42.
154. Albrecht M, Zitta K, Bein B, Wennemuth G, Broch O, Renner J, et al. Remote ischemic preconditioning regulates HIF-1α levels, apoptosis and inflammation in heart tissue of cardiosurgical patients: a pilot experimental study. Basic Research in Cardiology. 2013;108(1):314.
155. Trialists' Group TRP, Healy D, Khan W, Wong C, Moloney MC, Grace P, et al. Remote preconditioning and major clinical complications following adult cardiovascular surgery: systematic review and meta-analysis. International Journal of Cardiology. 2014;176(1):20-31.
156. Van den Akker EK, Hesselink DA, Manintveld OC, Lafranca JA, de Bruin RW, Weimar W, et al. Ischemic postconditioning in human DCD kidney transplantation is feasible and appears safe. Transplant International. 2014;27(2):226-34.
157. Zhao JJ, Xiao H, Zhao WB, Zhang XP, Xiang Y, Ye ZJ, et al. Remote Ischemic Postconditioning for Ischemic Stroke: A Systematic Review and Meta-Analysis of Randomized Controlled Trials. Chinese Medical Journal. 2018;131(8):956-65.
158. Hummitzsch L, Zitta K, Berndt R, Wong YL, Rusch R, Hess K, et al. Remote ischemic preconditioning attenuates intestinal mucosal damage: insight from a rat model of ischemia–reperfusion injury. Journal of Translational Medicine. 2019;17(1):136.
159. Miyake H, Koike Y, Seo S, Lee C, Li B, Ganji N, et al. The effect of pre-and post-remote ischemic conditioning reduces the injury associated with intestinal ischemia/reperfusion. Pediatric Surgery International. 2020;36(12):1437-42.
160. Holzner PA, Kulemann B, Kuesters S, Timme S, Hoeppner J, Hopt UT, et al. Impact of remote ischemic preconditioning on wound healing in small bowel anastomoses. World Journal of Gastroenterology: WJG. 2011;17(10):1308.
161. Yamashita N, Hoshida S, Taniguchi N, Kuzuya T, Hori M. A "second window of protection" occurs 24 h after ischemic preconditioning in the rat heart. Journal of Molecular and Cellular Cardiology. 1998;30(6):1181-9.
162. Hausenloy DJ, Yellon DM. The second window of preconditioning (SWOP) where are we now? Cardiovascular Drugs and Therapy. 2010;24(3):235-54.
163. Kin H, Zatta AJ, Lofye MT, Amerson BS, Halkos ME, Kerendi F, et al. Postconditioning reduces infarct size via adenosine receptor activation by endogenous adenosine. Cardiovascular Research. 2005;67(1):124-33.
164. Liu G, Thornton J, Van Winkle D, Stanley A, Olsson R, Downey J. Protection against infarction afforded by preconditioning is mediated by A1 adenosine receptors in rabbit heart. Circulation. 1991;84(1):350-6.
165. Davis JM, Gute DC, Jones S, Krsmanovic A, Korthuis RJ. Ischemic preconditioning prevents postischemic P-selectin expression in the rat small intestine. American Journal of Physiology-Heart and Circulatory Physiology. 1999;277(6):H2476-H81.
166. Penna C, Mancardi D, Rastaldo R, Losano G, Pagliaro P. Intermittent activation of bradykinin B2 receptors and mitochondrial KATP channels trigger cardiac postconditioning through redox signaling. Cardiovascular Research. 2007;75(1):168-77.
167. Wall TM, Sheehy R, Hartman JC. Role of bradykinin in myocardial preconditioning. Journal of Pharmacology and Experimental Therapeutics. 1994;270(2):681-9.
168. Schultz J, Rose E, Yao Z, Gross GJ. Evidence for involvement of opioid receptors in ischemic preconditioning in rat hearts. American Journal of Physiology - Heart and Circulatory Physiology. 1995;268(5):H2157-H61.
169. Zatta AJ, Kin H, Yoshishige D, Jiang R, Wang N, Reeves JG, et al. Evidence that cardioprotection by postconditioning involves preservation of myocardial opioid content and selective opioid receptor activation. American Journal of Physiology-Heart and Circulatory Physiology. 2008;294(3):H1444-H51.
170. You L, Li L, Xu Q, Ren J, Zhang F. Postconditioning reduces infarct size and cardiac myocyte apoptosis via the opioid receptor and JAK-STAT signaling pathway. Molecular Biology Reports. 2011;38(1):437-43.
171. Yang X-M, Proctor JB, Cui L, Krieg T, Downey JM, Cohen MV. Multiple, brief coronary occlusions during early reperfusion protect rabbit hearts by targeting cell signaling pathways. Journal of the American College of Cardiology. 2004;44(5):1103-10.
172. He B, Xiao J, Ren A-J, Zhang Y-F, Zhang H, Chen M, et al. Role of miR-1 and miR-133a in myocardial ischemic postconditioning. Journal of Biomedical Science. 2011;18(1):22.

173. Yin C, Salloum FN, Kukreja RC. A novel role of microRNA in late preconditioning: upregulation of endothelial nitric oxide synthase and heat shock protein 70. Circulation Research. 2009;104(5):572-5.
174. Tirpe AA, Gulei D, Ciortea SM, Crivii C, Berindan-Neagoe I. Hypoxia: overview on hypoxia-mediated mechanisms with a focus on the role of HIF genes. International Journal of Molecular Sciences. 2019;20(24):6140.
175. Semenza GL. Regulation of mammalian O2 homeostasis by hypoxia-inducible factor 1. Annual Review of Cell and Developmental Biology. 1999;15(1):551-78.
176. Saeedi BJ, Kao DJ, Kitzenberg DA, Dobrinskikh E, Schwisow KD, Masterson JC, et al. HIF-dependent regulation of claudin-1 is central to intestinal epithelial tight junction integrity. Molecular Biology of the Cell. 2015;26(12):2252-62.
177. Grenz A, Clambey E, Eltzschig HK. Hypoxia signaling during intestinal ischemia and inflammation. Curr Current Opinion in Critical Care. 2012;18(2):178-85.
178. Wiesener MS, Jürgensen JS, Rosenberger C, Scholze C, Hörstrup JH, Warnecke C, et al. Widespread, hypoxia-inducible expression of HIF-2α in distinct cell populations of different organs. The FASEB Journal. 2003;17(2):271-3.
179. Zhao H-X, Wang X-L, Wang Y-H, Wu Y, Li X-Y, Lv X-P, et al. Attenuation of myocardial injury by postconditioning: role of hypoxia inducible factor-1α. Basic Research in Cardiology. 2010;105(1):109.
180. Liu Y, Nie H, Zhang K, Ma D, Yang G, Zheng Z, et al. A feedback regulatory loop between HIF-1α and miR-21 in response to hypoxia in cardiomyocytes. FEBS letters. 2014;588(17):3137-46.
181. Feinman R, Deitch EA, Watkins AC, Abungu B, Colorado I, Kannan KB, et al. HIF-1 mediates pathogenic inflammatory responses to intestinal ischemia-reperfusion injury. American Journal of Physiology - Gastrointestinal and Liver Physiology. 2010;299(4):G833-G43.
182. Knudsen AR, Kannerup A-S, Grønbæk H, Andersen KJ, Funch-Jensen P, Frystyk J, et al. Effects of ischemic pre-and postconditioning on HIF-1α, VEGF and TGF-β expression after warm ischemia and reperfusion in the rat liver. Comparative Hepatology. 2011;10(1):3.
183. Wang P, Qi H, Sun C, He W, Chen G, Li L, et al. Overexpression of hypoxia-inducible factor-1alpha exacerbates endothelial barrier dysfunction induced by hypoxia. Cellular Physiology and Biochemistry. 2013;32(4):859-70.
184. Bauck A. G.; Grosche A.: Morton AJG, A. S.; Vickroy, T. W.; Freeman, D. E. Effect of lidocaine on in ammation in equine jejunum subjected to manipulation only and remote to intestinal segments subjected to ischemia. American Journal of Veterinary Research. 2017;78(8):977 - 89.
185. Kannan KB, Colorado I, Reino D, Palange D, Lu Q, Qin X, et al. Hypoxia-inducible factor plays a gut-injurious role in intestinal ischemia reperfusion injury. American Journal of Physiology - Gastrointestinal and Liver Physiology. 2011;300(5):G853-G61.
186. Lim SY, Davidson SM, Hausenloy DJ, Yellon DM. Preconditioning and postconditioning: the essential role of the mitochondrial permeability transition pore. Cardiovascular Research. 2007;75(3):530-5.
187. Pain T, Yang X-M, Critz SD, Yue Y, Nakano A, Liu GS, et al. Opening of mitochondrial KATP channels triggers the preconditioned state by generating free radicals. Circulation Research. 2000;87(6):460-6.
188. Cohen MV, Yang X-M, Downey JM. The pH hypothesis of postconditioning: staccato reperfusion reintroduces oxygen and perpetuates myocardial acidosis. Circulation. 2007;115(14):1895-903.
189. Whitley D, Goldberg SP, Jordan WD. Heat shock proteins: a review of the molecular chaperones. Journal of Vascular Surgery. 1999;29(4):748-51.
190. Oksala NK, Kaarniranta K, Tenhunen JJ, Tiihonen R, Heino A, Sistonen L, et al. Reperfusion but not acute ischemia in pig small intestine induces transcriptionally mediated heat shock response in situ. The Journal European Surgery 2002;34(6):397-404.
191. Fleming SD, Starnes BW, Kiang JG, Stojadinovic A, Tsokos GC, Shea-Donohue T. Heat stress protection against mesenteric I/R-induced alterations in intestinal mucosa in rats. Journal of Applied Physiology. 2002;92(6):2600-7.
192. Tons C, Klosterhalfen B, Klein HM, Rau HM, Anurov M, Oettinger A, et al. Induction of heat shock protein 70 (HSP70) by zinc bis (DL-hydrogen aspartate) reduces ischemic small-bowel tissue damage in rats. Langenbeck's Archives of Surgery. 1997;382(1):43-8.
193. Liao Y-F, Zhu W, Li D-P, Zhu X. Heme oxygenase-1 and gut ischemia/reperfusion injury: A short review. World Journal of Gastroenterology. 2013;19(23):3555.
194. Ibacache M, Sanchez G, Pedrozo Z, Galvez F, Humeres C, Echevarria G, et al. Dexmedetomidine preconditioning activates pro-survival kinases and attenuates regional ischemia/reperfusion injury in rat heart. Biochimica et Biophysica Acta (BBA)-Molecular Basis of Disease. 2012;1822(4):537-45.

195. Okada H, Kurita T, Mochizuki T, Morita K, Sato S. The cardioprotective effect of dexmedetomidine on global ischaemia in isolated rat hearts. Resuscitation. 2007;74(3):538-45.
196. Kopp V, Neudeck S, Pfarrer C, Kästner S, editors. Protective effects of dexmedetomidine-vatinoxan versus dexmedetomidine alone on intestinal ischemia-reperfusion injury in horses under genereal anaesthesia. World Congress of Veterinary Anesthesia; 2018; Venice.
197. Blikslager A, Roberts M, Gerard M, Argenzio R. How important is intestinal reperfusion injury in horses? Journal of the American Veterinary Medical Association (USA). 1997.
198. Kubes P, Hunter J, Granger DN. Ischemia/reperfusion-induced feline intestinal dysfunction: importance of granulocyte recruitment. Gastroenterology. 1992;103(3):807-12.
199. Blikslager AT, Roberts MC, Rhoads JM, Argenzio RA. Is reperfusion injury an important cause of mucosal damage after porcine intestinal ischemia? Surgery. 1997;121(5):526-34.
200. Gayle Jm, Jones SL, Argenzio RA, Blikslager AT. Neutrophils increase paracellular permeability of restituted ischemic-injured porcine ileum. Surgery. 2002;132(3):461-70.
201. Gonzalez LM, Moeser AJ, Blikslager AT. Animal models of ischemia-reperfusion-induced intestinal injury: progress and promise for translational research. American Journal of Physiology-Gastrointestinal and Liver Physiology. 2014;308(2):G63-G75.
202. Haessler R, Kuzume K, Chien GL, Wolff RA, Davis RF, Van Winkle DM. Anaesthetics alter the magnitude of infarct limitation by ischaemic preconditioning. Cardiovascular Research. 1994;28(10):1574-80.
203. Megison SM, Horton JW, Chao H, Walker PB. A new model for intestinal ischemia in the rat. Journal of Surgical Research. 1990;49(2):168-73.
204. Premen AJ, Banchs V, Womack WA, Kvietys PR, Granger DN. Importance of collateral circulation in the vascularly occluded feline intestine. Gastroenterology. 1987;92(5):1215-9.
205. Bean BP, Cohen CJ, Tsien RW. Lidocaine block of cardiac sodium channels. The Journal of General physiology. 1983;81(5):613.
206. Dzikiti T, Hellebrekers L, Van Dijk P. Effects of intravenous lidocaine on isoflurane concentration, physiological parameters, metabolic parameters and stress-related hormones in horses undergoing Surgery. Journal of Veterinary Medicine Series A. 2003;50(4):190-5.
207. Guschlbauer M, Slapa J, Huber K, Feige K. Lidocaine reduces tissue oedema formation in equine gut wall challenged by ischaemia and reperfusion. Pferdeheilkunde. 2010;26(4):531-4.
208. Cook VL, Jones Shults J, McDowell MR, Campbell NB, Davis JL, Marshall JF, et al. Anti-inflammatory effects of intravenously administered lidocaine hydrochloride on ischemia-injured jejunum in horses. American Journal of Veterinary Research. 2009;70(10):1259-68.
209. Canyon SJ, Dobson GP. Pretreatment with an adenosine A1 receptor agonist and lidocaine: a possible alternative to myocardial ischemic preconditioning. J Thorac Cardiovasc Surg. 2005;130(2):371-7.
210. Dobson GP, Jones MW. Adenosine and lidocaine: a new concept in nondepolarizing surgical myocardial arrest, protection, and preservation. The Journal of Thoracic and Cardiovascular Surgery. 2004;127(3):794-805.
211. Cook VL, Meyer CT, Campbell NB, Blikslager AT. Effect of firocoxib or flunixin meglumine on recovery of ischemic-injured equine jejunum. American Journal of Veterinary Research. 2009;70(8):992-1000.
212. Hall PA, Coates PJ, Ansari B, Hopwood D. Regulation of cell number in the mammalian gastrointestinal tract: the importance of apoptosis. Journal of Cell Science. 1994;107(12):3569-77.
213. Frisch SM, Francis H. Disruption of epithelial cell-matrix interactions induces apoptosis. The Journal of Cell Biology. 1994;124(4):619-26.
214. Sun X-M, MacFarlane M, Zhuang J, Wolf BB, Green DR, Cohen GM. Distinct caspase cascades are initiated in receptor-mediated and chemical-induced apoptosis. Journal of Biological Chemistry. 1999;274(8):5053-60.
215. Alnemri ES, Livingston DJ, Nicholson DW, Salvesen G, Thornberry NA, Wong WW, et al. Human ICE/CED-3 protease nomenclature. Cell. 1996;87(2):171.
216. Nuñez G, Benedict MA, Hu Y, Inohara N. Caspases: the proteases of the apoptotic pathway. Oncogene. 1998;17(25):3237-45.
217. Liu X, Zou H, Slaughter C, Wang X. DFF, a heterodimeric protein that functions downstream of caspase-3 to trigger DNA fragmentation during apoptosis. Cell. 1997;89(2):175-84.
218. Grossmann J, Mohr S, Lapetina EG, Fiocchi C, Levine AD. Sequential and rapid activation of select caspases during apoptosis of normal intestinal epithelial cells. American Journal of Physiology - Gastrointestinal and Liver Physiology. 1998;274(6):G1117-G24.

219.Grossmann J, Artinger M, Grasso AW, Kung H-J, Schölmerich J, Fiocchi C, et al. Hierarchical cleavage of focal adhesion kinase by caspases alters signal transduction during apoptosis of intestinal epithelial cells. Gastroenterology. 2001;120(1):79-88.

220.Cardone MH, Roy N, Stennicke HR, Salvesen GS, Franke TF, Stanbridge E, et al. Regulation of cell death protease caspase-9 by phosphorylation. Science. 1998;282(5392):1318-21.

221.Gold R, Schmied M, Giegerich G, Breitschopf H, Hartung H, Toyka K, et al. Differentiation between cellular apoptosis and necrosis by the combined use of in situ tailing and nick translation techniques. Laboratory investigation; Journal of Technical Methods and Pathology. 1994;71(2):219-25.

222.Al-Lamki R, Skepper J, Loke Y, King A, Burton G. Apoptosis in the early human placental bed and its discrimination from necrosis using the in-situ DNA ligation technique. Human reproduction. 1998;13(12):3511-9.

223.Didenko VV, Ngo H, Baskin DS. Early necrotic DNA degradation: presence of blunt-ended DNA breaks, 3' and 5' overhangs in apoptosis, but only 5' overhangs in early necrosis. The American Journal of Pathology. 2003;162(5):1571-8.

224.Lindeström L-M, Ekblad E. Structural and neuronal changes in rat ileum after ischemia with reperfusion. Digestive Diseases and Sciences. 2004;49(7-8):1212-22.

225.Mei F, Guo S, He YT, Zhu J, Zhou DS, Niu JQ, et al. Apoptosis of interstitial cells of Cajal, smooth muscle cells, and enteric neurons induced by intestinal ischemia and reperfusion injury in adult guinea pigs. Virchows Archives 2009;454(4):401-9.

226.Rivera LR, Thacker M, Pontell L, Cho H-J, Furness JB. Deleterious effects of intestinal ischemia/reperfusion injury in the mouse enteric nervous system are associated with protein nitrosylation. Cell and Tissue Research. 2011;344(1):111-23.

227.Pontell L, Sharma P, Rivera LR, Thacker M, Tan YH, Brock JA, et al. Damaging effects of ischemia/reperfusion on intestinal muscle. Cell and Tissue Research. 2011;343(2):411-9.

228.Blikslager AT, Bowman K, Levine J, Bristol D, Roberts M. Evaluation of factors associated with postoperative ileus in horses: 31 cases (1990-1992). Journal of the American Veterinary Medical Association. 1994;205(12):1748-52.

229.Lisowski Z, Pirie R, Blikslager A, Lefebvre D, Hume D, Hudson N. An update on equine post-operative ileus: Definitions, pathophysiology and management. Equine Veterinary Journal. 2018;50(3):292-303.

230.Kalff JC, Carlos TM, Schraut WH, Billiar TR, Simmons RL, Bauer AJ. Surgically induced leukocytic infiltrates within the rat intestinal muscularis mediate postoperative ileus. Gastroenterology. 1999;117(2):378-87.

231.Little D, Tomlinson JE, Blikslager AT. Post operative neutrophilic inflammation in equine small intestine after manipulation and ischaemia. Equine Veterinary Journal. 2005;37(4):329-35.

232.Turner JR. Intestinal mucosal barrier function in health and disease. Nature Reviews Immunology. 2009;9(11):799-809.

233.McKenzie JA, Ridley AJ. Roles of Rho/ROCK and MLCK in TNF-α-induced changes in endothelial morphology and permeability. Journal of Cellular Physiology. 2007;213(1):221-8.

234.Suenaert P, Bulteel V, Lemmens L, Noman M, Geypens B, Van Assche G, et al. Anti-tumor necrosis factor treatment restores the gut barrier in Crohn's disease. The American Journal of Gastroenterology. 2002;97(8):2000-4.

235.Madara JL, Stafford J. Interferon-gamma directly affects barrier function of cultured intestinal epithelial monolayers. The Journal of Clinical Investigation. 1989;83(2):724-7.

236.Kucharzik T, Walsh SV, Chen J, Parkos CA, Nusrat A. Neutrophil transmigration in inflammatory bowel disease is associated with differential expression of epithelial intercellular junction proteins. The American Journal of Pathology. 2001;159(6).

237.Sugiyama S, Okada Y, Sukhova GK, Virmani R, Heinecke JW, Libby P. Macrophage myeloperoxidase regulation by granulocyte macrophage colony-stimulating factor in human atherosclerosis and implications in acute coronary syndromes. The American journal of pathology. 2001;158(3):879-91.

238.Bos A, Wever R, Roos D. Characterization and quantification of the peroxidase in human monocytes. Biochimica et Biophysica Acta - Enzymology. 1978;525(1):37-44.

239.Yui S, Nakatani Y, Mikami M. Calprotectin (S100A8/S100A9), an inflammatory protein complex from neutrophils with a broad apoptosis-inducing activity. Biological and Pharmaceutical Bulletin. 2003;26(6):753-60.

240.Grosche A, Morton AJ, Polyak MM, Matyjaszek S, Freeman DE. Detection of calprotectin and its correlation to the accumulation of neutrophils within equine large colon during ischaemia and reperfusion. Equine Veterinary Journal. 2008;40(4):393-9.

241. Rötting AK, Freeman DE, Constable PD, Eurell JAC, Wallig MA. Effects of ischemia and reperfusion on eosinophilic accumulation and distribution in mucosa of equine jejunum and colon. American Journal of Veterinary Research. 2016;77(5):534-9.

242. Kemper D, Perkins G, Schumacher J, Edwards J, Valentinen B, Divers T, et al. Equine lymphocytic-plasmacytic enterocolitis: a retrospective study of 14 cases. Equine Veterinary Journal. 2000;32(S32):108-12.

243. Yagmurdur H, Ozcan N, Dokumaci F, Kilinc K, Yilmaz F, Basar H. Dexmedetomidine reduces the ischemia-reperfusion injury markers during upper extremity surgery with tourniquet. The Journal of Hand Surgery. 2008;33(6):941-7.

244. Arslan M, Metin Çomu F, Küçük A, Öztürk L, Yaylak F. Dexmedetomidine protects against lipid peroxidation and erythrocyte deformability alterations in experimental hepatic ischemia reperfusion injury. Libyan Journal of Medicine. 2012;7(1):18185.

245. Tasdogan M, Memis D, Sut N, Yuksel M. Results of a pilot study on the effects of propofol and dexmedetomidine on inflammatory responses and intraabdominal pressure in severe sepsis. Journal of Clinical Anesthesia. 2009;21(6):394-400.

246. Venn R, Bryant A, Hall GM, Grounds R. Effects of dexmedetomidine on adrenocortical function, and the cardiovascular, endocrine and inflammatory responses in post-operative patients needing sedation in the intensive care unit. British Journal of Anaesthesia. 2001;86(5):650-6.

247. Lai Y-C, Tsai P-S, Huang C-J. Effects of dexmedetomidine on regulating endotoxin-induced up-regulation of inflammatory molecules in murine macrophages. Journal of Surgical Research. 2009;154(2):212-9.

248. Poffers M, Buhne N, Herzog C, Thorenz A, Chen R, Guler F, et al. Sodium Channel Nav1.3 Is Expressed by Polymorphonuclear Neutrophils during Mouse Heart and Kidney Ischemia In Vivo and Regulates Adhesion, Transmigration, and Chemotaxis of Human and Mouse Neutrophils In Vitro. Anesthesiology. 2018;128(6):1151-66.

249. Schmidt W, Schmidt H, Bauer H, Gebhard MM, Martin E. Influence of lidocaine on endotoxin-induced leukocyte-endothelial cell adhesion and macromolecular leakage in vivo. Anesthesiology: The Journal of the American Society of Anesthesiologists. 1997;87(3):617-24.

250. Cook VL, Neuder LE, Blikslager AT, Jones SL. The effect of lidocaine on in vitro adhesion and migration of equine neutrophils. Veterinary Immunology and Immunopathology. 2009;129(1-2):137-42.

251. Grimm KA, Lamont LA, Tranquilli WJ, Greene SA, Robertson SA. Veterinary anesthesia and analgesia: the fifth edition of Lumb and Jones: John Wiley & Sons; 2015.

252. Kishikawa H, Kobayashi K, Takemori K, Okabe T, Ito K, Sakamoto A. The effects of dexmedetomidine on human neutrophil apoptosis. Biomedical Research. 2008;29(4):189-94.

253. Chen Y, Lee S-H, Tsai Y-H, Tseng S-H. Ischemic preconditioning increased the intestinal stem cell activities in the intestinal crypts in mice. Journal of Surgical Research. 2014;187(1):85-93.

254. Wan D, Zhang Z, Yang H. Cardioprotective effect of miR-214 in myocardial ischemic postconditioning by down-regulation of hypoxia inducible factor 1, alpha subunit inhibitor. Cellular and Molecular Biology. 2015;61(2):1.

11. Acknowledgements

First of all, I would like to thank Prof. Dr. Sabine Kästner for her advice and support in her role as my main supervisor. I am very grateful for the connections she made for me, for her scientific views, and for the space she provided to make my own decisions, yet always being available for consultation.

I would like to thank Prof. Dr. Marion Hewicker-Trautwein for her guidance in dealing with a variety of immunohistochemical challenges and for her accessible manner. I am also grateful for the supervision provided by Prof. Dr. Christiane Pfarrer, whose positive encouragement has meant a great deal. Furthermore, I would like to thank my external supervisor Prof. Dr. Anja Kipar for her knowledgeable advice and contributions to the discussion of the project.

Aside from my supervision group, several other institutes got on board, resulting in a multidisciplinary mix. First, I would like to thank Prof. Dr. Gerhard Breves and Prof. Dr. Gemma Mazzuoli-Weber from the Institute for Physiology and Cell Biology for their contributions and contagious enthusiasm. Furthermore, I would like to express my gratitude to Prof. Dr. Maren von Köckritz-Blickwede and Nicole de Buhr, PhD from the Department of Biochemistry for their welcoming "can-do" attitude and professional guidance.

In addition to the scientific input from the professors of the different institutes, I am grateful for the practical and technical support I received from many other members of these departments. For this I would like to thank Kerstin Rohn from the Institute of Pathology, Silke Akhdar from the Department of Biochemistry, Doris Voigtländer and Marion Langeheine from the Institute for Anatomy, and Marion Burmester and Nadine Schnepel from the Institute for Physiology and Cell Biology.

Furthermore, I would like to thank Henri Schulte and Dr. Christina Brandenberger from the Institute of Functional and Applied Anatomy of the Hannover Medical School for the digitalisation of the countless histology slides. I am grateful for all the statistical advice provided by Dr. Karl Rohn, ever so patient. I would also like to express my gratitude to the Hannover Graduation School for facilitating this PhD Program and for the involved organisation and coordination by Prof. Dr. Beatrice Behrens, Dr. Tina Selle, and Tanja Czeslik.

From the Clinic for Horses, I would like to thank everyone who was involved in the care for the horses and the execution of the experimental trials. More specifically, I am grateful to Dr. Stephan Neudeck and Dr. Lara Twele for their important role in the organisation and execution of the experiments, and to my predecessors Dr. Kathrin König and Veronika Kopp for showing me the way in the world of 'Winterversuchen'. Furthermore, I would like to thank Jane Kühn and Anna-Lena Schubert for their excellent assistance during the experimental trials. Many of my dear colleagues, who I cannot all mention personally, have offered a listening ear and crucial advice in dealing with all kinds of issues, and have provided great assistance in my everlasting German language struggles. Special thanks are addressed to Dr. Alexander Schwieder, for always having my back in the clinic when patient care and research turned out to be incompatible.

Finally, I am very grateful for the people in my life who did not have much to do with the contents of this work, yet have everything to do with me being where I am now. I would like to thank my family, especially my parents, who have always encouraged me to follow my passion, and who have given me confidence and a sense of determination. My dearest friends have played an important part in maintaining some form of work-life balance, respecting my busy schedule and listening to my endless work stories, but also keeping me from becoming too narrow minded. Ultimately, my most heartfelt thank you is for my partner Joost Ernst, for walking next to me every single step of the way.

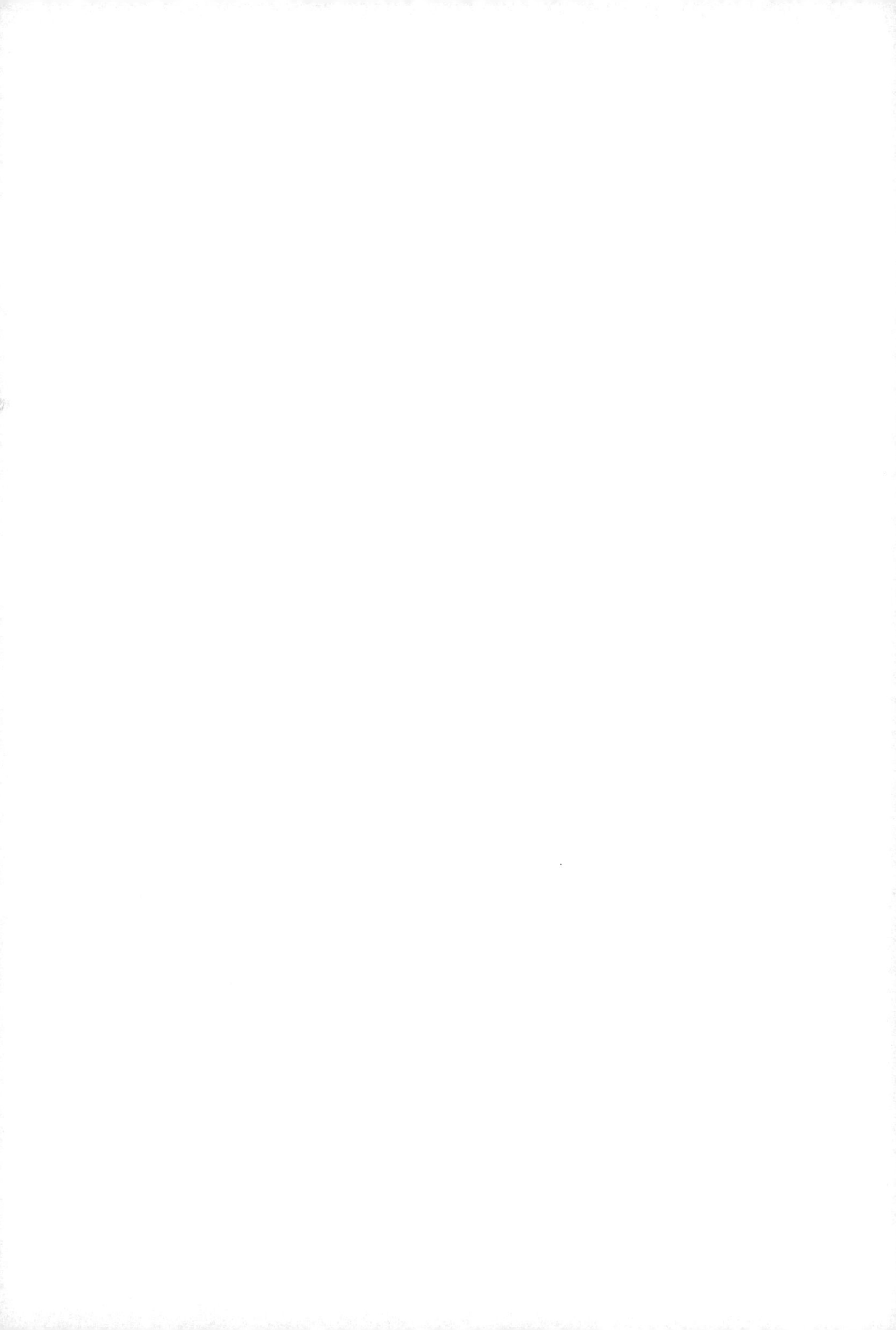

www.ingramcontent.com/pod-product-compliance
Ingram Content Group UK Ltd.
Pitfield, Milton Keynes, MK11 3LW, UK
UKHW022000190726
13853UKWH00004B/1646

9 783736 974333